CO.

Laboratory and Diagnostic Testing in Psychiatry

American Psychiatric Press

CONCISE GUIDES

Robert E. Hales, M.D.
Series Editor

CONCISE GUIDE TO

Laboratory and Diagnostic Testing in Psychiatry

Richard B. Rosse, M.D.
Assistant Professor of Psychiatry

Alexis A. Giese, M.D.
Instructor in Psychiatry

Stephen I. Deutsch, M.D., Ph.D.
Chief, Psychiatry Service
Associate Professor of Psychiatry

John M. Morihisa, M.D.
Professor of Psychiatry

Washington Veterans Administration Medical Center
Georgetown University School of Medicine
Washington, D.C.

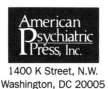

American Psychiatric Press, Inc.

1400 K Street, N.W.
Washington, DC 20005

First Edition   04 03 02 01   13 12 11 10

The paper used in this publication meets the minimum require-
ments of American National Standard for Information Sciences—Permanence of Paper for Printed Library Materials,
ANSI Z39.48-1984.   ∞

Library of Congress Cataloging-in-Publication Data

Concise guide to laboratory and diagnostic testing in psychiatry/
   Richard B. Rosse . . . [et al.].
       p.   cm.—(Concise guides/American Psychiatric Press)
   Includes bibliographies and index.
   ISBN 0-88048-333-4 (alk. paper)
   1. Diagnosis, Laboratory—Handbooks, manuals, etc.
2. Mental illness—Diagnosis—Handbooks, manuals, etc.
I. Rosse, Richard B. II. Series: Concise guides (American Psychiatric Press)
       [DNLM: 1. Diagnosis, Laboratory. 2. Mental Disorders—
diagnosis. WM 141 C744]
RC473.L32C66   1989
616.89′075—dc19
DNLM/DLC
for Library of Congress   89-3
                                                               CIP

CONTENTS

APPENDIX C: LIST OF SELECTED ABBREVIATIONS   137

INTRODUCTION

to the *American Psychiatric Press Concise Guides*

The *American Psychiatric Press Concise Guides* series provides, in a most accessible format, practical information for psychiatrists—and especially for psychiatry residents and medical students—working in such varied treatment settings as inpatient psychiatry services, outpatient clinics, consultation-liaison services, and private practice. The *Concise Guides* are meant to complement the more detailed information to be found in lengthier psychiatry texts.

The *Concise Guides* address topics of greatest concern to psychiatrists in clinical practice. The books in this series contain a detailed Table of Contents, along with an index, tables, and charts, for easy access; and their size, designed to fit into a lab coat pocket, makes them a convenient source of information. The number of references has been limited to those most relevant to the material presented.

For psychiatrists in both general hospital settings and in outpatient practice, the appropriate use of laboratory and diagnostic test evaluations is a critical component of their practice. The authors of this volume, Drs. Richard Rosse, Alexis Giese, Stephen Deutsch, and John Morihisa, are all very experienced, biologically oriented psychiatrists who work at the Washington Veterans Administration Medical Center, one of the Veterans Administration's flagship hospitals. All are affiliated with the Department of Psychiatry at the Georgetown University School of Medicine.

The authors have focused their efforts in providing practical and clinically relevant information. They have organized their book into eight chapters. They begin by writing an overview of basic strategies that should be used in applying laboratory testing in psychiatric practice. They then proceed to focus on five general laboratory evaluation areas of relevance and importance to psychiatrists: endocrine, hematologic, biochemical, immunologic, and toxicology assessments. Their discussion of tests is succinct, yet well documented. For instance, in Chapter 2, which discusses endocrine evaluations, they emphasize why the laboratory assessment of thyroid function is important and outline some of the most common thyroid tests: serum triiodothyronine, thyroxine, thyroid-stimulating hormone, T_3 resin uptake, free T_4, free thyroxine index, antithyroglobulin antibodies, and antithyroid microsomal antibodies. In addition to describing the tests, they discuss how to interpret the results and when to order more sophisticated or supplementary tests, such as the thyrotropin-releasing hormone stimulation test. The remainder of Chapter 2 is devoted to other common endocrinologic tests of clinical relevance to psychiatrists, such as the dexamethasone suppression test.

The other chapters of the book have a similar comprehensive yet abbreviated format. The chapters are well written and full of important information that residents and practitioners will need. Their particular evaluations are especially helpful. They put in perspective for psychiatrists when to order tests and how to approach interpreting the results.

This is a book that psychiatrists and physicians in other specialties will turn to frequently to answer questions or to obtain additional important information. The authors included a number of tables that assist the reader in remembering key points. Their appendixes are particularly outstanding. Appendix A gives formulas for calculating sensitivity, specificity, and positive and negative predictive power. Appendix B is a marvelous addition to the book. As the authors emphasize, consensus of what test to order for selected psychiatric conditions varies. However, they have meticulously reviewed the current psychiatric literature and have summarized in Appendix B their recommended workup for selected conditions: alcohol abuse and dependence, anorexia nervosa, atypical psychosis, bulimia, dementia, a general psychiatric patient admission battery, and the neuroleptic malignant syndrome. Appendix B is particularly helpful in that it provides concrete guidelines to follow in ensuring that all appropriate tests have been ordered. Whenever appropriate, the authors have included references to document their recommendations. Appendix C is a useful list of abbreviations that are commonly used in clinical practice.

Since I had the pleasure of reading and rereading this book in manuscript form, I have found myself already using it frequently in my own clinical work. I believe that the readers of this volume will find it to be a helpful and an authoritative manual. The authors are to be congratulated for their outstanding scholarship and ability to condense a great amount of material into this *Concise Guide*. Psychiatrists, and especially psychiatric residents and medical students, should find the *Concise Guide to Laboratory and Diagnostic Testing in Psychiatry* to be a valuable addition to their medical library.

Robert E. Hales, M.D.
Series Editor
American Psychiatric Press Concise Guides

PREFACE

The goal of this book is to assist the psychiatric clinician in improving some of his or her diagnostic skills, specifically in the area of the laboratory evaluation of the psychiatric patient. This concise handbook, however, should be thought of only as a *guide* to some of the clinical utility that certain laboratory and other diagnostic examinations have for the psychiatrist; consultation with longer, more in-depth medical textbooks will often be necessary. The psychiatrist is also encouraged to ask questions of the clinicians in the laboratories that they use. These laboratory-based clinicians are often a useful resource for up-to-date information on laboratory testing and can provide the psychiatrist with suggestions that apply to the needs of particular patients and the demands of the test methodology used by the specific laboratory. The psychiatrist should not hesitate to confer with these laboratory physicians with questions about the proper performance or interpretation of certain laboratory tests. Similarly, consultation with other medical specialists is often required when the psychiatrist is considering other diagnostic tests for their patients, including consultation with radiologists about computed tomographic and magnetic resonance imaging studies, with cardiologists regarding electrocardiogram interpretation, and with neurologists when certain neurologic evaluations (e.g., electroencephalogram, lumbar puncture) are involved.

The reader should note that there is incomplete consensus about some of the concepts presented in this book; when possible, different opinions have been briefly outlined. References have been provided to allow the interested reader to investigate particular areas further. As time goes on, it is certain that various ideas presented will be subject to change as new data are reported. It is hoped that this book will be useful to the clinician in providing a foundation for evaluating some of these changes.

Finally, this book should not be seen as a ticket to the runaway use of laboratory and diagnostic testing in psychiatry. It has been said that many tests performed in clinical medicine today do not substantially contribute to improved patient care and result in the waste of precious health-care dollars. Indeed, it is often useful for the clinician to have a price list for the laboratory and diagnostic tests that they order for their patients (and for which their patients will have to pay); such a price list should help to inhibit the clinician's ordering of whimsical and adventure-some tests. It is hoped that this book will help the psychiatrist to make intelligent choices about laboratory and diagnostic tests and help to maximize use of the results obtained from these tests.

Richard B. Rosse, M.D.
Alexis A. Giese, M.D.
Stephen I. Deutsch, M.D., Ph.D.
John M. Morihisa, M.D.

ACKNOWLEDGMENTS

The authors would like to thank Elvira Grant and Denise M. Reeves for their diligent and careful attention to the preparation of the manuscript. We would also like to extend our appreciation to Robert Hales, M.D., Series Editor of the *Concise Guides* series, for giving us the opportunity to write this book.

INTRODUCTION

■ THE GROWING ROLE OF LABORATORY AND DIAGNOSTIC TESTING IN PSYCHIATRY

The use of laboratory and other diagnostic tests in psychiatry is increasing for a number of reasons. There is a growing awareness of the need for a basic medical evaluation of psychiatric patients to rule out possible underlying medical conditions that might be contributing to the patient's psychiatric presentation. Generally, the use of these tests is based on clues provided by the history, review of systems, and physical examination.

With psychiatrists' increasing use of certain psychotropic medications (e.g., lithium, tricyclic antidepressants, anticonvulsants), there has been a growing appreciation of the usefulness of monitoring blood levels of these medications and their metabolites to guide therapy and to minimize adverse reactions.

With the illicit substance abuse epidemic currently manifest in our country, there is an increasing need for psychiatric clinicians to be able to detect those patients whose psychiatric conditions might be affected by drug abuse. Alcohol and drug abuse histories obtained from patients are often unreliable. In the context of drug abuse treatment, the laboratory has also been used to monitor the effectiveness of the therapy and to help motivate the patient to comply with abstinence.

A growing awareness of the biologic aspects of psychiatric illness has led to a search for biologic "markers" that could help identify certain psychiatric disorders and guide treatment. Although no biologic marker has yet been established as having clear clinical utility, research in this area continues.

Finally, the medical training of psychiatrists has made them accustomed to utilizing laboratory and diagnostic tests in their evaluation and treatment of patients. As physicians, it is important to be able to order these tests appropriately and to interpret them accurately. Psychiatrists need to be aware of the limitations of the tests they employ and to be realistic about what they can expect of these tests. It is also important to recognize when one has reached the limits of one's own expertise in a certain area and know when it is most appropriate to consult nonpsychiatric medical colleagues.

■ AN OVERVIEW OF STRATEGIES FOR LABORATORY TESTING IN PSYCHIATRY

NONSELECTIVE VERSUS SELECTIVE APPROACHES TO THE ROUTINE SCREENING BATTERY

No consensus exists as to which tests would make up the most appropriate screening battery for the psychiatric patient. One way to divide some of the differences of opinion about routine laboratory testing strategies is to separate the differences into the "nonselective" and "selective" schools. The nonselective ("shotgun") approach recommends a broad screening battery as part of the search for potential underlying medical disorders. The selective approach encourages a narrower selection of routine tests and emphasizes the thoughtful use of supplemental tests ordered on the basis of clinical relevance. Physicians advocating a selective approach typically express the belief that it is more cost-effective than a nonselective strategy and that selective approaches do not compromise patient care (1).

UTILIZATION OF LABORATORY AND DIAGNOSTIC TESTS IN PSYCHIATRY

At this time, the clinician will need to use his or her clinical judgment in deciding which tests to utilize in a particular situation. This judgment should be grounded on group consensus on diagnostic testing strategies in psychiatry and on research evaluations of clinical utility (1). Unfortunately, complete consensus on these matters does not exist in the literature, and "usual practice" for particular problems or types of patients varies somewhat.

The clinician should realize that usually the best diagnostic evaluation consists of a good history and physical and mental status examinations by a psychiatrist with some understanding of the psychiatric manifestations of medical illness. Unfortunately, the medical history is often a neglected part of the psychiatric examination. In Appendix B, some sample screening batteries for different categories of patients can be found; however, the physician's choice of diagnostic tests should be individualized, based on the patient's history and physical and mental status examinations. Overtesting, besides being expensive, results in unnecessary patient discomfort, inconvenience, and the possibility that false-positive tests will lead to further unnecessary testing. Conversely, undertesting also has its hazards; certain underlying medical illnesses responsible for a psychiatric presentation might go unrecognized when proper diagnostic tests are not obtained (2). Computer programs are under development to help the physician order laboratory tests that have the highest probability of showing abnormal results for a particular patient (3).

RESEARCH EVALUATIONS

Research psychiatrists have been increasingly accumulating evidence for subtle neurophysiologic dysfunction in many psychiatric patients. Efforts are being made to quantitate some of these abnormalities. Although there are some biologic measures utilized as supplemental tests by some clinicians, the vast majority of these biologic evaluations should be seen as research tools that require further clarification of their clinical utility.

■ REFERENCES

1. Dolan JG, Mushlin AI: Routine laboratory testing for medical disorders in psychiatric inpatients. Arch Intern Med 1985; 145:2085–2088
2. National Institutes of Health Consensus Development Panel: Differential diagnosis of dementing disease. National Institutes of Health Consensus Development Conference Statement 1987; 6:1–9
3. Tierney WM, McDonald CJ, Hui SL, et al: Computer predictions of abnormal test results: effects on outpatient testing. JAMA 1988; 259:1194–1198

■ ADDITIONAL READINGS

Giannini AJ, Black HR, Goettsche RL: Psychiatric, Psychosomatic and Somatopsychic Disorders Handbook. Garden City, NY, Medical Examination Publishing, 1978

Hales RE: The diagnosis and treatment of psychiatric disorders in medically ill patients. Milit Med 1986; 151:587–595

Hall RCW, Beresford TP: Laboratory evaluation of newly admitted psychiatric patients, in Handbook of Psychiatry Diagnostic Procedures, vol 1. Edited by Hall RCW, Beresford TP. New York, SP Medical and Scientific Books, 1984

Hall RCW, Popkin MK, Devaul RA, et al: Physical illness presenting as psychiatric disease. Arch Gen Psychiatry 1978; 35:1315–1320

Hoffman RS, Koran LM: Detecting physical illness in patients with mental disorders. Psychosomatics 1984; 25:654–660

2 ENDOCRINE EVALUATIONS OF POTENTIAL RELEVANCE TO PSYCHIATRISTS

Endocrinopathies can have psychiatric manifestations. The endocrinopathy can present with clear physical signs and symptoms of the disorder or be manifest only by psychiatric, behavioral, or cognitive abnormalities. The psychiatrist should be knowledgeable about the laboratory and diagnostic tests available to help detect what are often subtle endocrine disturbances.

■ THYROID FUNCTION

Numerous psychiatric conditions have been associated with thyroid dysfunction, including depression, psychosis, panic, anxiety, hypomania, dementia, and delirium. Many clinicians recommend that some type of thyroid function testing be done routinely with psychiatric patients who have not had recent thyroid testing to detect possible thyroid illness that might be contributing to or causing a patient's psychiatric condition. However, some clinicians restrict their thyroid function testing to those patients who manifest clear signs or symptoms of possible thyroid disease. Figure 2-1 outlines an algorithm proposed by Raj and Sheehan (1) that applies to a laboratory evaluation of thyroid function in a psychiatric patient.

Major reasons for obtaining thyroid function tests in psychiatric patients include identification of those psychiatric patients who 1) might need thyroid hormone replacement or supplementa-

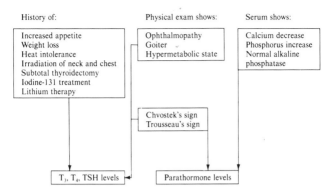

FIGURE 2-1. **Strategy for the evaluation of thyroid disorder**
Adapted from Raj A, Sheehan DV: Medical evaluation of panic attacks. J Clin Psychiatry
1987; 48:309–313. With permission from publisher. Copyright 1987 Physicians Postgraduate
Press.

tion, 2) might need treatment for hyperthyroidism, and 3) might
be experiencing thyrotoxicity secondary to lithium therapy.

There is no complete consensus as to which thyroid function
tests should be routinely ordered. For instance, some clinicians
might just order a serum thyroxine (T_4). Other clinicians order a
thyroid battery consisting of thyroid-stimulating hormone (TSH)
radioimmunoassay (RIA), T_4, and triiodothyronine resin uptake
(T_3RU). Still others might also include a serum triiodothyronine
(T_3) or even measures of antithyroid antibodies. Most recently,
the TSH as measured by the sensitive immunoradiometric assay
(IRMA) has been recommended as a useful screening test for
suspected thyroid disease (see Figure 2-2) (2).

OUTLINE OF SOME THYROID FUNCTION TESTS

Serum triiodothyronine (T_3), typically measured by RIA,
measures both protein-bound and unbound T_3, i.e., total T_3. T_3 is
useful in detecting hyperthyroidism. Isolated elevations of T_3
(with normal T_4) can be seen in "T_3 toxicosis." Although it has
been reported that depressed patients as a group tend to have

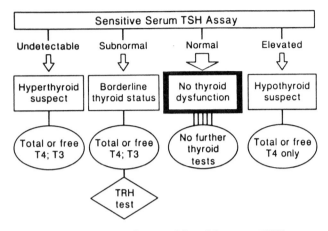

FIGURE 2-2. **Algorithm for use of "sensitive serum TSH assay" (TSH-IRMA) in the laboratory evaluation of thyroid function**

Using the sensitive TSH assay, the TSH-IRMA would typically be the only test needed unless other signs or symptoms suggesting thyroid dysfunction were present. T_4 = thyroxine; T_3 = triiodothyronine; TRH test = thyrotropin releasing hormone (stimulation) test. From Klee GG, Hay ID: Assessment of sensitive thyrotropin assays for an expanded role in thyroid function testing: proposed criteria for analytic performance and clinical utility. J Clin Endocrinol Metab 1987; 64:461–471. Reproduced with permission from publisher. Copyright 1987 The Endocrine Society.

evidence of decreased thyroid function (e.g., lower T_3 levels than normal controls), the thyroid function tests are typically not out of the "normal ranges" established for most laboratories (3). Serum T_3 can be low in both hypothyroidism and nonthyroidal illness. Usually the reverse T_3 (rT_3) is also low in hypothyroidism, but typically is high in nonthyroidal illness, secondary to a decrease in the conversion of T_4 to T_3, with an increase in rT_3. Reverse T_3 values increase with age, probably due to a decrease in the peripheral conversion of T_4 and T_3. Interestingly, Orsulak et al. (3) speculated that patients with depression convert less T_4 to T_3 and instead shunt a greater proportion of T_4 to the biologically inactive rT_3.

Serum thyroxine (T_4), also usually measured by RIA and useful in the detection of hyperthyroidism, measures both protein-bound and unbound (i.e., total) T_4. As with most laboratory values, normal values can vary depending on the measurement methodology utilized and the population that was used to determine the "normal" values.

Serum thyroid-stimulating hormone (TSH), also known as thyrotropin, can be measured by RIA and, more recently, by immunoradiometric assay (IRMA). For many years the TSH-RIA has been important in the diagnosis of primary hypothyroidism, which is characterized by an increased concentration of TSH. On *rare* occasions, an increased TSH level can be seen in hyperthyroidism (the result of a TSH-secreting pituitary tumor). Generally, low TSH-RIA values have been considered nondiagnostic and can be consistent with hyperthyroidism, pituitary hypothyroidism, or even euthyroid status. However, the newer, more sensitive TSH-IRMA is helpful in the laboratory evaluation of hypo- and hyperthyroidism (see Figure 2-2). Unlike with the TSH-RIA, with the TSH-IRMA it is possible to distinguish euthyroid from hyperthyroid patients, largely eliminating the need for the thyrotropin-releasing hormone (TRH) stimulation test in the diagnosis of hyperthyroidism. Detectable amounts of TSH by IRMA can be found in patients with hypothyroidism due to pituitary or hypothalamic disease. Therefore, patients with this rare form of hypothyroidism (2° hypothyroidism) can conceivably be missed using the TSH-IRMA. Medically hospitalized and unstable patients have been reported to have a high rate of abnormal TSH-IRMA results due to nonthyroidal illness or therapy with dopamine or glucocorticoids; less controversial is the use of the sensitive TSH-IRMA in stable, ambulatory patients with intact hypothalamic-pituitary function.

T_3 resin uptake (T_3RU) is an indirect measure of thyroid binding protein. Normal values can vary slightly, depending on the specific methodology used. Elevations can reflect such conditions as hyperthyroidism or disease states causing protein depletion (e.g., nephrotic syndrome, liver disease, malnutrition). Decreased T_3RU can be seen in hypothyroidism or conditions causing increases in patient serum protein available for in vitro radioactive T_3 binding (e.g., pregnancy), and hence, less radioactive T_3 is available to bind to the added hormone-binding resin used in the T_3RU assay. The numeric value of the resin uptake is inversely proportional to plasma binding; lower thyroid binding

protein or thyroxine-binding globulin (TBG) levels are reflected by increased T_3RU values, and vice versa. Typically, T_4 and T_3RU are both increased in hyperthyroidism and both decreased in hypothyroidism. When the T_4 and T_3RU are abnormal in opposite directions (i.e., T_4 is decreased while the T_3RU is increased or vice versa), a protein-binding abnormality is suggested. A direct and specific test for abnormal T_4 binding not affected by other serum proteins is available as thyroxine-binding globulin (TBG-RIA). TBG should not be confused with *thyroglobulin*; the latter is a storage prohormone for T_4 and T_3 normally found in the thyroid, but that can enter the bloodstream in various thyroid disease states including thyroiditis and certain thyroid cancers.

Free T_4 (fT_4) measures unbound T_4. T_4 bioactivity resides in the T_4 fraction that is unbound ("free"). fT_4 can be measured directly either by using an equilibrium dialysis method or by RIA kits that measure fT_4. This test, like T_3RU, helps correct for protein-binding changes of T_4. This is becoming a very popular screening test for thyroid dysfunction.

The free thyroxine index (FTI), sometimes referred to as T_7 or T_{12}, is the result of the serum T_4 value multiplied by the T_3RU. The FTI calculation often helps increase the sensitivity of the T_4 value in detecting hypo- or hyperthyroidism (by correcting for the effects of thyroid binding protein changes on the T_4 assays). Note that changes in thyroid binding proteins typically have opposite effects on the T_4 and T_3RU; hence, the use of the FTI helps to cancel the effects an altered protein status might have on the T_4.

Antithyroglobulin antibodies and antithyroid microsomal antibodies (or thyroid antimicrosomal antibodies) can be found in Hashimoto's thyroiditis (HT), atrophic thyroiditis, or symptomless autoimmune thyroiditis (SAT). Shader and Greenblatt (4) commented that HT can be found in 1 to 2 percent of autopsies of the general population and that most patients with HT are clinically euthyroid, although there may be a nontender goiter causing slight discomfort or dysphagia. A patient with histologic confirmed HT without serologic evidence of thyroid antibodies has been described, suggesting that HT can exist as an organ-restricted autoimmune disorder (5). Antithyroid antibodies are also often elevated in patients with Grave's disease. Some clinical investigators have recommended that patients with elevated TSH measures (baseline or in response to TRH) should perhaps be evaluated for the presence of antithyroid antibodies.

Gold et al. (6) questioned whether antithyroid antibody–positive patients with SAT are indeed "symptomless" and wondered what the role of this disorder might be for many patients with affective disorders. The presence of antithyroid antibodies has been reported to occur with a greater than expected frequency in patients with affective symptoms, patients who are dexamethasone suppression test (DST) nonsuppressors, and patients with a "chronic infectious mononucleosis" type picture characterized by persistent weakness, fatigue, anxiety, or depression. The presence of antithyroid antibodies in a population of psychiatric patients being treated for major mood disorders (bipolar disorders) was reported to be 21.7 percent versus a prevalence of antithyroid antibodies in the general population of approximately 10 percent (7). Indeed, some psychiatric clinicians are utilizing measures of thyroid autoantibodies as part of their thyroid evaluation of some psychiatric patients, especially those with affective symptoms. It has also been suggested that the presence of baseline antithyroid antibodies might be predictive of future lithium-induced hypothyroidism. Further study will be needed to define clearly the prognostic and therapeutic meaning of thyroid autoantibodies in psychiatric patients.

INTERPRETATION OF THYROID FUNCTION TEST RESULTS

Table 2-1 outlines some typical results of thyroid function tests in various conditions. Various thyroid function test abnormalities have been reported in a significant minority (around 10 percent) of newly hospitalized psychiatric patients. The abnormal findings in many of these patients reportedly became spontaneously normal with time.

Interpretation of thyroid function tests can be quite difficult and often requires the assistance of a medical specialist (e.g., internist or endocrinologist). It should be remembered that alterations in thyroid function tests are not always a reflection of true thyroid disease, but can be a result of metabolic derangements seen in other medical conditions or due to certain medication effects.

TABLE 2-1. **Laboratory Evaluation of Thyroid Function in Various Thyroid Disorders**

Physiologic State	Serum T_4 (Thyroxine)	Serum T_3 (Triiodo-thyronine)	Resin T_3 (Triiodothyro-nine Uptake)
Hyperthyroidism, untreated	High	High	High
Hyperthyroidism, T_3 toxicosis	Normal	High	Normal
Hypothyroidism, untreated	Low	Low	Low
Euthyroid, on iodine	Normal	Normal	Normal
Euthyroid, on endogenous thyroid hormone	High, on T_4 Low, on T_3	High, on T_3 Normal, on T_4	Normal
Euthyroid, on estrogen	High	High	Low
Euthyroid, on phenytoin	Low	Low	High

Note. From Berkow R (ed): The Merck Manual of Diagnosis and Therapy, 15th ed., p. 1037. Used with permission. Copyright 1987 Merck and Co., Inc.

THE THYROTROPIN-RELEASING HORMONE STIMULATION TEST

The thyrotropin-releasing hormone stimulation test (TRHST) was originally developed by endocrinologists to evaluate the functioning of the hypothalamic-pituitary-thyroid (HPT) axis. Release of TRH from the hypothalamus results in the secretion of TSH from the anterior pituitary gland. TSH then acts on the thyroid gland to stimulate the release of thyroid hormone. In the TRHST, TRH is administered exogenously through an intravenous cannula, and serum thyrotropin (TSH) levels are followed. In the hands of psychiatrists, the TRHST has been used 1) in the workup of possible "subclinical" hypothyroidism in the depressed patient and 2) as a potential biologic marker of major depression in euthyroid patients.

METHOD

In a commonly described version of the test, blood is initially drawn for a TSH assay, and then 500 μg of TRH is given intravenously over a one- to three-minute duration while the patient is at bed rest (8, 9). This test is commonly performed around 9:00 AM. Note that bolus injections of TRH between 200 and 600 μg have been described (10). A blood sample for TSH determination is then taken at 30 minutes post-TRH administration; blood for TSH samples can also be drawn at 60 and/or 90 minutes post-TRH injection. However, the TSH peak tends to occur approximately 20 to 30 minutes after the TRH infusion, and many clinicians will just sample 30 minutes post-TRH administration (10). A delta TSH is determined by subtracting the baseline TSH from the peak TSH after TRH stimulation. Side effects of the TRH infusion can include transient autonomic symptoms (e.g., tachycardia, an urge to urinate). In a normal individual, the TRH challenge causes the serum TSH to increase about 5 to 25 μIU/ml within 15 to 20 minutes after the TRH injection. The serum TSH then returns to baseline over about two hours postinjection.

THE TRHST IN THE DETECTION OF HYPOTHYROIDISM

A TRHST can help determine whether or not a patient is hypothyroid and can be of assistance in "grading" a patient's hypothyroidism. Three grades of hypothyroidism have been described: Grade I—overt hypothyroidism, with clear historical, physical, and laboratory evidence of hypothyroidism; Grade II—"mild" hypothyroidism, where the T_4 is normal but the TSH is elevated; and Grade III—"subclinical" hypothyroidism, where the T_4 and TSH are normal and only the TRHST is abnormal. Antithyroid antibodies are reportedly more common in all these grades of hypothyroidism than in the euthyroid, normal population. Note that clinical depression reportedly can be seen in any of these grades of hypothyroidism.

Generally, patients with primary hypothyroidism have an exaggerated TSH response to TRH challenge, whereas the hyperthyroid patient is more likely to have a flat serum TSH response (i.e., the change in TSH is ≤ 5 to 7 μIU/ml). However, a blunted TSH response is not diagnostic of hyperthyroidism. Hyperthyroidism should also be associated with other thyroid function test abnormalities (e.g., elevated T_4 and T_3). Note that physiologic conditions that would tend to inhibit the pituitary release of TSH (e.g., starvation, high circulating levels of dopamine or steroids) might result in blunted TSH responses to TRH challenge.

Targum et al. (11) suggested that treatment-resistant depressed patients with an augmented TSH response (defined by that group as $>30 \mu IU/ml$), with otherwise-normal thyroid indices, might benefit from adjunctive thyroid hormone added to their antidepressant regimen. These are patients who are perhaps approaching a hypothyroid status (i.e., Grade III hypothyroidism).

THE TRHST AS BIOLOGIC MARKER OF DEPRESSION

The TRHST has also been proposed as a potential biologic marker of affective disorder (8, 9). Most investigators feel comfortable using the TRHST this way as a research tool, but consider its clinical potential as requiring further investigative clarification.

A blunted TSH response (typically characterized as a delta TSH ≤ 5 to $7 \mu IU/ml$) has been reported in many patients with major affective disorders. Such a blunted TSH response has been reported to occur about 25 to 30 percent of the time in patients with major depression (8, 9). Note, however, that blunted TSH responses have also been reported in many patients with alcoholism (even after prolonged abstinence), bulimia, borderline personality, and panic disorder. Interestingly, these are illnesses that have been hypothesized as somehow related to affective disorders (12).

Some investigators have also proposed that a positive TRHST is related to the severity of the depression and a history of violent suicide attempts. The utility of the TRHST to help evaluate severity of depression or suicide potential or predict or assess treatment response is an important research question.

POTENTIAL CONFOUNDING VARIABLES IN USING THE TRHST AS A BIOLOGIC MARKER FOR DEPRESSION

Factors that have been reported to affect the delta TSH and to confound the interpretation of the TRHST include thyroid diseases, other endocrine diseases, hepatic or renal failure, advanced age, weight loss, alcohol intoxication or withdrawal, and treatment with steroids, diphenylhydantoin, carbamazepine, estrogens, and lithium. Recent cocaine use has also been reported to cause abnormal TRHST results.

■ ADRENAL DISEASE

As with thyroid disease, adrenal dysfunction has been associated with a wide range of psychiatric disturbances, including mood disorders (e.g., depression, mania), anxiety disorders, psychosis, delirium, and dementia. Hence, the psychiatrist should be aware of some of the laboratory tests available to test for adrenal disease. Some of these tests (e.g., the cosyntropin stimulation test) might best be ordered and performed while in consultation with an appropriate specialist (e.g., internist, endocrinologist).

None of these tests are typically ordered by psychiatrists on a routine basis. They are ordered as supplemental tests when adrenal disease is suspected. Their use as biologic markers of psychiatric illness (e.g., depression) is controversial.

OUTLINE OF SOME LABORATORY TESTS FOR ADRENAL DISEASE

Plasma cortisol detects abnormalities in cortisol secretion from the adrenal glands. Low plasma cortisol (typically less than 5 μg/dl) suggests Addison's disease. Plasma cortisols above 20 μg/dl suggest Cushing's disease. Plasma cortisol, as measured by RIA or competitive protein binding, measures both free and protein-bound cortisol, i.e., total cortisol levels. Only unbound cortisol is active at the tissue and cellular levels. Measures of free cortisol are not currently available for routine clinical use. The usefulness of plasma free cortisol as a marker of depression is under investigation.

Abnormalities of cortisol secretion, specifically cortisol hypersecretion, have been frequently noted in patients with affective disorders (13). Along with this hypercortisolism, severe depression has been associated with a possible loss of the normal diurnal variation of cortisol secretion (10) and is the basis of the diurnal cortisol test (DCT). Interestingly, a lower prevalence of hypercortisolism has been reported in patients with schizophrenia than in patients with major depression (14).

Urinary free cortisol, urinary 17-hydroxycorticosteroids, and urinary 17-ketosteroids detect hyperadrenocorticism. Elevated urinary free cortisol (UFC), sometimes in the range found in Cushing's disease, has been reported in depressed patients, but these findings have not always been replicated. Furthermore, in depressed patients, UFC decreases have been described as often paralleling clinical improvement. Elevated urinary 17-hydroxycorticosteroid levels (collected over a 24-hour period) have been used by some as a suicide predictor in high-risk patients; however, low or normal values do not necessarily imply low risk for suicide.

Urinary metanephrine, urinary vanillylmandelic acid (VMA), and urinary catecholamines are used in the workup of patients suspected of having pheochromocytoma. Most pheochromocytomas can be diagnosed by measuring these in 24-hour urine collections.

Plasma catecholamines (epinephrine and norepinephrine) are useful in the workup of pheochromocytoma, especially after paroxysmal spells of autonomic hyperexcitability (e.g., as manifested by a period of hypertension or tachycardia). Figure 2-3 outlines the laboratory and other diagnostic test evaluations of the patient with suspected pheochromocytoma proposed by Raj and Sheehan (2). On another note, researchers have reported that decreases in plasma *homovanillic acid* (a dopamine metabolite) levels in schizophrenic patients treated with antipsychotics have correlated with improvement in psychosis ratings.

The *cosyntropin (Cortrosyn) stimulation test* is used by endocrinologists in the evaluation of adrenal insufficiency. Cosyntropin is a synthetic adrenocorticotropic hormone (ACTH) preparation. This test has also been utilized by some research psychiatrists as a marker of major depression. A *corticotropin-releasing hormone (CRH) stimulation test* has also been used by research psychiatrists; a blunting of ACTH responses in depressed patients has been reported.

THE DEXAMETHASONE SUPPRESSION TEST AS A BIOLOGIC MARKER OF DEPRESSION

The *dexamethasone suppression test (DST)* is used by endocrinologists in the workup of Cushing's disease and by some

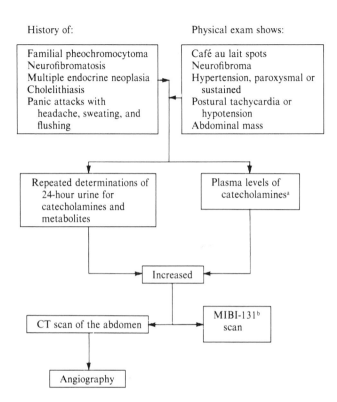

History of:

- Familial pheochromocytoma
- Neurofibromatosis
- Multiple endocrine neoplasia
- Cholelithiasis
- Panic attacks with headache, sweating, and flushing

Physical exam shows:

- Café au lait spots
- Neurofibroma
- Hypertension, paroxysmal or sustained
- Postural tachycardia or hypotension
- Abdominal mass

Repeated determinations of 24-hour urine for catecholamines and metabolites

Plasma levels of catecholamines[a]

Increased

CT scan of the abdomen

MIBI-131[b] scan

Angiography

FIGURE 2-3. **Laboratory and diagnostic test strategy for the evaluation of pheochromocytoma**

Adapted from Raj A, Sheehan DV: Medical evaluation of panic attacks. J Clin Psychiatry 1987; 48:309–313. With permission from publisher. Copyright 1987 Physicians Postgraduate Press. [a]Blood sample should be drawn from the patient after 30 minutes of bed rest, from a previously inserted indwelling catheter. [b]Scintigraphic imaging after injection of meta-iodobenzyl guanidine labeled with iodine-131, which helps locate catecholamine-secreting tumors.

psychiatrists as a possible biologic marker for major depression. For psychiatrists, the DST has been proposed as a way of detecting subtle abnormalities of the hypothalamic-pituitary-adrenal axis that have been hypothesized to be present in patients with endogenous depression. This test has been proposed as having both diagnostic and prognostic significance in depressed patients. The DST has been the subject of hundreds of research papers that have appeared in the psychiatric literature. However, there is no general agreement as to its clinical utility. The American Psychiatric Association (APA) Task Force on the Use of Laboratory Tests in Psychiatry (15) has outlined some of the uses and limitations of the DST in clinical psychiatry, some of which are listed in Table 2-2.

DST METHODOLOGY

The DST is performed over a two-day period. In a commonly described version of the DST (10), the patient has a blood sample drawn for a baseline cortisol at about 11:00 PM on the first day of the test, after which the patient receives 1 mg of dexamethasone orally. Some clinicians draw the baseline pre-dexamethasone cortisol at 8:00 AM on that first day of the test.

After the patient receives 1 mg of dexamethasone at or

TABLE 2-2. **APA Task Force Recommendations for the Dexamethasone Suppression Test (DST)**

1. Usefulness not high when a patient is either very likely or very unlikely to have a major affective disorder. In these cases, clinical judgment is probably sufficient.

2. A positive DST may encourage some patients to accept recommended somatic treatment and therefore might be useful in patients who would otherwise resist these necessary treatment modalities.

3. A negative test should *not* discourage somatic treatment if appropriate.

4. The DST may be useful in certain ambiguous situations (e.g., psychotic affective disorder versus acute schizophrenic illness).

5. After apparent recovery, persistent nonsuppression of the DST warrants close follow-up. However, the converse is not necessarily true (i.e., patients whose DST normalizes still require careful follow-up as clinically indicated).

Note. American Psychiatric Association Task Force on the Use of Laboratory Tests in Psychiatry: The dexamethasone suppression test: an overview of its current status in psychiatry. Am J Psychiatry 1987; 144:1253–1262. Copyright 1987 American Psychiatric Association.

around 11:00 PM on the first day of the test, blood cortisols are usually drawn over the next 24 hours, typically at 8:00 AM, 4:00 PM, and 11:00 PM of the following day (day 2). Some variance in blood sample collection times (e.g., one-hour variances) are generally acceptable. Some time variance (e.g., 30 minutes) either way for dexamethasone administration is also typically tolerated.

The procedure outlined above can be implemented fairly easily in an inpatient setting; it is generally less easily done for outpatients. For convenience to outpatients, often only an afternoon (e.g., 4:00 PM) blood sample is obtained. However, decreasing the number of post-dexamethasone blood cortisols that are drawn reportedly does result in a modest loss of test sensitivity (15).

DEFINITION OF ABNORMAL DST RESULTS

The DST is usually considered abnormal, or positive, if the post-dexamethasone serum cortisol levels equal or exceed about 5 μg/dl (138 nmol/liter in SI units); however, this cutoff point can vary slightly from one laboratory to another. Also, different methods for measuring plasma or serum cortisol levels are used by different hospitals and commercial laboratories. The two most commonly used methodologies are RIA and competitive protein-binding assay (PBA). The APA Task Force (15) recommends that each laboratory regularly standardize its procedures to maintain assay quality and to define the appropriate criterion level for cortisol. Recent studies outlined in the APA Task Force report that tested commercially available cortisol RIA have yielded inconsistent assay values for the same sample and have found that even the same assay method could be inconsistent over time. Because normal values between laboratories are variable and because plasma cortisol concentrations close to 5 μg/dl are often not carefully standardized, the APA Task Force (15) recommended that post-dexamethasone serum or plasma cortisol levels between 4 and 7 μg/dl "be interpreted cautiously."

LIMITATIONS OF THE DST IN PSYCHIATRY

Although there is controversy concerning the clinical value of the DST, some psychiatrists have included it in their evaluation of patients with an affective disorder (or a possible affective "component" to their psychiatric disorder). Some specific limitations to the use of the DST include

1. A reported sensitivity in the range of only 45 percent (perhaps higher in psychotic affective disorder).
2. A reported specificity in healthy controls around 90 percent, but a much lower specificity when the DST is used in patients with psychiatric disorders other than depression. Unfortunately, the test is most commonly utilized in the lower specificity condition; that is, the test is utilized to help differentiate between depression and other psychiatric disorders, not to help differentiate depression from no psychiatric condition.
3. The clinician should be aware of the fact that the possibility of significant artifactual contamination exists, including various drugs (e.g., barbiturates, carbamazepine, phenytoin), endocrine abnormalities (e.g., Cushing's disease, pregnancy, diabetes mellitus), and other medical conditions (15).

THE UTILITY OF DST RESULTS

Overall, there does not appear to be a clinical situation where a DST result would, or should, significantly affect treatment decisions, overriding good clinical judgment. The usefulness of what was called by some "psychiatry's sed rate" seems to be primarily as a research tool. In the clinical situation, an abnormal DST might help to increase the probability of a particular patient having a diagnosis of an affective disorder, or at least some affective component to his or her psychiatric presentation. An abnormal DST has also been proposed as possibly predicting a good response to somatic treatment (10). A normal DST result in a psychiatric patient is not felt to have specific clinical utility. Additionally, the DST does not appear to be appropriate for routine screening of all psychiatric patients (16). Finally, it has been suggested that the DST may prove useful in helping to predict relapse in some patients treated for depression (17), although the evidence at this time is not conclusive on this matter (15).

THE DEXAMETHASONE SUPPRESSION INDEX

Arana et al. (18) reported enhancement of DST diagnostic

utility for depression by use of a "dexamethasone suppression index," which is the product of the patient's serum cortisol and serum dexamethasone levels expressed in SI units ([nmol/liter]^2). The use of such an index helps to control for those patients with low plasma dexamethasone levels, which could presumably lead to spurious DST nonsuppression. According to Arana et al. (18), the DST test performance, based on analyses of sensitivity, specificity, and predictive power, was improved when the dexamethasone suppression index was utilized. They reported that at a criterion level of 400 [nmol/liter]^2, the 8:00 AM calculation for the dexamethasone suppression index achieved a specificity of 100 percent and sensitivity of 69 percent. The dexamethasone suppression index should not be confused with the cortisol suppression index (CSI) described by Bernstein et al. (19). The CSI is a ratio of pre- to post-dexamethasone cortisol concentration, with ratios less than 4 often regarded as significant for nonsuppression. These other ways of expressing the DST result require further study.

ALTERNATIVE METHODOLOGIES FOR PERFORMING THE DST

The DST method described above requires the patient to submit to anywhere from two to four venipunctures over about a 24-hour period. This requires the use of a trained phlebotomist and exposes the patient to some pain and inconvenience. Some alternative methodologies involving less pain and more convenience have been studied. Some very preliminary work has suggested that salivary cortisol determinations can be used in place of the serum cortisol assays (20). Martin et al. (20) used salivary cortisols below 90 ng/dl as their criteria for nonsuppression. Using a criteria of cortisol nonsuppression in serum of 5 μg/dl, they reported that 29 of 30 patients had similar findings in both saliva and serum. A kit for the salivary DST is commercially available. More research will be needed to clearly establish its reliability and clinical utility.

■ OTHER FORMS OF ENDOCRINE DYSFUNCTION

Besides thyroid and adrenal disorders, a number of other endocrine dysfunctions have been associated with psychiatric disorders. These include disorders of the pancreas, as well as problems related to the secretion of antidiuretic hormone (ADH), parathyroid hormone, growth hormone (GH), prolactin, testosterone, and estrogen. Additionally, knowledge about the reproductive status of the female psychiatric patient is important for the psychiatrist because this can affect certain diagnostic and treatment decisions.

OUTLINE OF SOME LABORATORY TESTS OF PANCREATIC FUNCTION

The major role of the pancreas is the regulation of blood glucose levels.

Fasting blood sugar (FBS) is useful in the evaluation of diabetes mellitus. Very high blood sugars (hyperglycemia) can be associated with delirium (especially in the context of diabetic ketoacidosis). Low blood sugars (hypoglycemia) have been associated with psychiatric symptoms such as delirium, depression, agitation, anxiety, and panic attacks.

Postprandial blood glucose is used by some clinicians in the evaluation of patients complaining of symptoms suggestive of "reactive hypoglycemia." Symptoms can include fatigue, nervousness, tremor, tachycardia, sweating, and hunger; these symptoms are typically reported three to five hours after a meal. Note that the great majority of patients complaining of reactive hypoglycemia and presenting with these symptoms have normal postprandial blood sugars after meals and even during symptomatic periods. Some investigators have recommended the use of the term *idiopathic postprandial syndrome* in patients complaining of postmeal symptoms of reactive hypoglycemia in the absence of documentable hypoglycemia. Blood for postprandial glucose determination is commonly drawn two hours after a meal or after ingestion of a glucose solution containing about 75 g of glucose. General use of this test is currently not recommended for the evaluation of reactive hypoglycemia.

The *glucose tolerance test* (GTT) is used in the detection of either decreased glucose tolerance (e.g., as in diabetes mellitus and Cushing's disease) or increased glucose tolerance (e.g., as in Addison's disease, hypothyroidism, or hypopituitarism). The oral GTT is commonly used in the evaluation of patients with some symptoms or complications associated with diabetes mellitus, but who do not have FBSs above 140 mg/dl. It is also commonly used to detect gestational diabetes in pregnant women (21). Psychoactive medications known to decrease glucose tolerance include haloperidol, phenothiazines, chlorprothixene, lithium carbonate, and tricyclic antidepressants (TCAs).

Formerly, the GTT was also commonly used in the diagnosis of reactive hypoglycemia (thought caused by "overproduction" of insulin in response to glucose load during meals in certain sensitive patients). However, low glucose levels (e.g., less than 50 mg/dl) have been found to be almost as common in asymptomatic patients as in those who experience symptoms thought related to hypoglycemia (22). The use of the GTT specifically in the evaluation of reactive hypoglycemia is currently being discouraged. The *mixed meal test* (MMT) is sometimes used instead of the GTT in the diagnosis of reactive hypoglycemia. The MMT better replicates the patient's actual dietary experience. With the MMT, reactive hypoglycemia in the absence of a pancreatic pathologic lesion (e.g., an insulinoma) is uncommon.

HYPOGLYCEMIA IN PSYCHIATRIC DISORDERS

Hypoglycemia can at times be the cause of psychiatric symptomatology. McFarland et al. (22) described some causes of hypoglycemia, including 1) physiologic (e.g., as many as a third of athletes who exercise to exhaustion have blood glucose levels less than 45 mg/dl), 2) exogenously induced (e.g., by oral hypoglycemic agents, insulin injection), and 3) secondary to medical conditions (e.g., insulinoma, chronic renal failure, myxedema, pituitary or adrenal insufficiency). Figure 2-4 outlines an algorithm proposed by Raj and Sheehan (1) for the evaluation of hypoglycemia in psychiatric patients. In addition to the strategy proposed in Figure 2-3, glucose determinations can be performed during a suspected hypoglycemic episode. Hypoglycemia can present with a number of different mental status changes, including anxiety, panic attacks, delirium, confusion, or agitation (sometimes severe). Boyle et al. (23) reported an average glycemic threshold for symptoms of hypoglycemia to be 2.9 ± 0.1 mmol/liter (53 ± 2 mg/dl) in subjects without diabetes; and a symptomatic glycemic threshold to be 4.3 ± 0.3

History of:

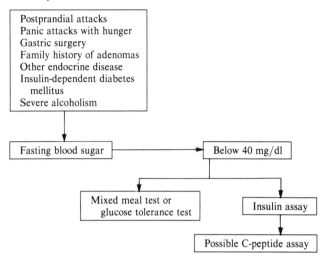

| Postprandial attacks |
| Panic attacks with hunger |
| Gastric surgery |
| Family history of adenomas |
| Other endocrine disease |
| Insulin-dependent diabetes mellitus |
| Severe alcoholism |

Fasting blood sugar → Below 40 mg/dl

Mixed meal test or glucose tolerance test

Insulin assay

Possible C-peptide assay

FIGURE 2-4. Strategy for the evaluation of hypoglycemia
Adapted from Raj A, Sheehan DV: Medical evaluation of panic attacks. J Clin Psychiatry 1987; 48:309–313. With permission from publisher. Copyright 1987 Physicians Postgraduate Press.

mmol/liter (78 ± 5 mg/dl) in patients with poorly controlled diabetes. Blood for glucose determinations can be obtained either by venipuncture or fingerstick; chemstrips or electronic glucose monitors can be used to get a blood glucose reading from a fingerstick.

In the presence of significant hypoglycemia in a psychiatric patient, consultation with a medical specialist is useful and should include the investigation of possible hyperinsulinism. Further laboratory workup might involve the simultaneous determination of plasma glucose, insulin, and C-peptide levels. In endogenous hyperinsulinism (e.g., secondary to an insulinoma), both plasma insulin and C-peptide levels are generally high. A low blood level of C-peptide might suggest an intentional (i.e., factitious) induction of hypoglycemia by insulin injection. (Note that C-peptide is the part of the proinsulin molecule that is removed when insulin is secreted from the pancreas and therefore should be found with insulin in equal amounts.) Factitious hypoglycemia secondary to oral antidiabetic agents (e.g., sulfonylureas) would typically show elevated insulin and C-peptide levels.

OTHER TESTS USED TO ASSESS PANCREATIC FUNCTION

A discussion of serum amylase and lipase can be found in Chapter 4. For an evaluation of possible pancreatic carcinoma (e.g., sometimes presenting to a psychiatrist in a patient complaining of back or abdominal pain or in a patient with depression), diagnostic tests employed include pancreatic ultrasound, an abdominal computed tomography (CT) scan, and needle or open biopsy of the pancreas. Other evidence of pancreatic dysfunction can sometimes also be seen in patients with pancreatic carcinoma.

■ MEASURES USED TO EVALUATE ANTIDIURETIC HORMONE SECRETION AND FUNCTIONING

Serum ADH is also known as vasopressin; decreased ADH levels are suggestive of central diabetes insipidus (DI).

Urine osmolality is useful in the evaluation of polyuric conditions (e.g., DI) and in hyper- or hyponatremic states. Urine osmolality is decreased in DI and in patients with polydipsia and normal kidney function without uncontrolled diabetes.

Plasma osmolality is useful in the evaluation of polyuric conditions (e.g., DI) and in hyper- or hyponatremic states. Plasma osmolality is typically increased in DI and can be decreased in patients with water intoxication secondary to psychogenic polydipsia.

EVALUATION OF DIABETES INSIPIDUS

The two major forms of DI are nephrogenic and pituitary (central) DI.

NEPHROGENIC DI

Two forms of nephrogenic DI exist. They are

1. An *inherited*, X-linked condition. Affected males appear to be completely unresponsive to ADH. The disorder begins in infancy.
2. An *acquired* form, such as lithium-induced DI. Lithium decreases the kidney tubules' sensitivity to ADH. Patients on lithium with excessive urine outputs (e.g., exceeding 4 liters per day) are vulnerable to severe orthostasis or vascular collapse.

PITUITARY, OR ADH-SENSITIVE, DI

Here, the insulting lesions (e.g., gliosis, tumors, stroke) are located in the brain (i.e., hypothalamus or pituitary). In patients with ADH-sensitive DI, polyuria decreases with exogenously administered ADH. This forms the basis of the vasopressin challenge test used to help differentiate between nephrogenic and pituitary DI. Pituitary DI can also be divided into primary (or idiopathic) DI, which is present from infancy, and acquired DI, which results from various pathologic lesions of the hypothalamus or pituitary (e.g., head trauma, posthypophysectomy) or is related to other cranial insults where there has been either pituitary or hypothalamic injury.

SYNDROME OF INAPPROPRIATE SECRETION OF ANTIDIURETIC HORMONE

The *syndrome of inappropriate secretion of antidiuretic hormone* (SIADH) is characterized by hyponatremia secondary to increased retention of body fluid resulting from excessive secretion of ADH. It has been associated with certain medical conditions (e.g., bronchogenic carcinoma, tuberculosis, pneumonia, porphyria, acute leukemia, myxedema, brain tumors, infections of the central nervous system, head trauma, and stroke) as well as certain medications (e.g., carbamazepine, phenothiazines, chlorpropamide, potassium-depleting diuretics, and antitumor drugs such as vincristine and cyclophosphamide).

This condition is relevant to psychiatrists for three reasons:

1. Hyponatremia can be associated with mental status changes (usually of a delirious nature). These changes might be confused with a worsening of a patient's psychiatric condition. Severe hyponatremia can result in seizures and coma.

2. As alluded to before, there have been anecdotal reports of SIADH associated with the administration of various psychotropics including antipsychotics such as phenothiazines and butrophenones, TCAs, monoamine oxidase inhibitors (MAOIs), and carbamazepine (24). SIADH has also been associated with cigarette smoking, which can be excessive in certain chronic psychiatric patients (25).

3. Rarely, SIADH has been reported in patients with psychosis (e.g., schizophrenia and recurrent affective disorders), even when these patients are off all psychiatric medications (26). In these cases, the SIADH has been postulated to be triggered by certain neuroendocrine changes possibly brought about through the emotional stress of psychosis. Also, some lowered intrinsic set point for the release of ADH in these patients has been postulated (27). SIADH can also be seen in the context of psychogenic polydipsia. The polydipsia combined with some degree of SIADH further predisposes the patient to the development of serious hyponatremia, although psychogenic polydipsia by itself can cause water intoxication and hyponatremia. However, patients with polydipsia alone reportedly do not generally experience substantial hyponatremia. It is when the compulsive water drinking is combined with increased circulating ADH that the patient seems at greatest risk for severe drops in serum sodium. Indeed, psychosis, polydipsia, and SIADH can be associated as a triad (28).

LABORATORY MONITORING OF SIADH

SIADH is accompanied by hyponatremia, abnormally low serum osmolality, and high urine osmolality, all in the presence of otherwise-normal endocrine, renal, hepatic, and cardiovascular functioning. Fluid and electrolyte balance in patients with SIADH can be monitored by evaluating serum electrolytes, especially serum sodium, as well as serum and urine osmolalities. These values also need to be closely followed to measure the effectiveness of the treatment interventions (e.g., discontinuation or lowering of the offending medication, fluid restriction, administration of demeclocycline). SIADH should be suspected when there is a combination of hyponatremia and an inappropriately concentrated urine (high specific gravity, high urine osmolality).

SIADH is a condition for which a careful evaluation for the primary cause of the disorder is indicated. This can frequently be assisted by consultation with a knowledgeable internist or endocrinologist.

■ OTHER ENDOCRINE LABORATORY EVALUATIONS

Parathormone (or parathyroid hormone) is involved in regulating blood calcium and phosphorous levels. Dysregulation has been associated with a wide variety of organic mental disorders. An indication for obtaining a serum parathormone level might include finding abnormal calcium and/or phosphorus blood levels. A strategy for deciding whether to measure a parathormone level in a psychiatric patient can be found in Figure 2-1.

Serum growth hormone (GH) is used in the evaluation of hyperpituitary (e.g., gigantism and acromegaly) and hypopituitary (e.g., Simmonds' disease) syndromes. Follicle-stimulating hormone (FSH), luteinizing hormone (LH), and TSH are typically low in patients with panhypopituitarism (Simmonds' disease).

Psychiatric researchers have been investigating the potential usefulness of serum GH responses to such pharmacologic challenges as dopamine, apomorphine, dextroamphetamine, clonidine, benzodiazepines, and insulin-induced hypoglycemia. Results include reports of blunted GH responses to insulin-induced hypoglycemia in patients with depressive disorders (10) and augmented GH responses to apomorphine challenge in patients with schizophrenia and patients with Schenedarian first-rank symptoms (29).

Serum prolactin levels can be used in the evaluation of patients on antipsychotics with galactorrhea. Antipsychotics block dopamine receptors in the pituitary and cause subsequent prolactin synthesis and release, an effect that seems particularly pronounced in women. These elevated prolactin levels can cause galactorrhea in some patients. Interestingly, the atypical antipsychotic clozapine reportedly does not induce significant serum prolactin elevations. Serum prolactin levels should normalize with the discontinuation of the offending medication. Another potential use of serum prolactin is after a seizurelike event; lack of rise in serum prolactin is viewed by some as suggestive of pseudoseizure (30). Also, prolactin challenge tests (e.g., apomorphine, TRH, or methadone challenge) have been studied by various psychiatric researchers. Finally, elevated prolactin levels have been reported in patients during withdrawal from heavy cocaine use.

Serum testosterone levels are part of the organic evaluation of the impotent patient. Note that normal values are usually different for adolescent and adult males and females. Typically, FSH and LH are also measured as part of an impotence workup. Decreases in serum testosterone can be seen in men with decreased sexual drive.

Measurement of serum testosterone levels is frequently a part of the evaluation of other medical conditions, including testosterone-producing (virilizing) tumors, Klinefelter's syndrome, cryptorchidism, primary and secondary hypogonadism, and Kallmann's syndrome. Serum testosterone and LH levels have been noted to decrease in male sex offenders treated with medroxyprogesterone acetate. (Liver transaminase elevations can also be seen in patients treated with this medication.)

Serum estradiol, the most active of the endogenous estrogens, is commonly used in evaluating menstrual and infertility problems. In males, estradiol levels can be used in the evaluation of gynecomastia or feminizing states (e.g., possibly secondary to estrogen-producing tumors).

Pregnancy tests are classified here as endocrine evaluations because most pregnancy tests currently employed are immunologically based evaluations of the pregnancy hormone, human chorionic gonadotropin (HCG). HCG can be measured in urine or blood samples by various methodologies. Pregnancy can usually be detected by two weeks after an expected menstrual period. Pregnancy status may be important for the clinical psychiatrist for the following reasons:

1. Certain psychotropic medications (e.g., lithium) can adversely affect the developing fetus. The clinician and patient need to

be aware of the childbearing status so that appropriate informed treatment decisions can be made. For example, it is frequently recommended that the use of lithium be avoided during the first trimester of pregnancy if at all possible.

2. Pregnancy can change the patient's renal clearance of lithium.
3. Pregnancy can result in an exacerbation of a patient's psychiatric condition.

Hormonal changes have been suspected as being involved in premenstrual syndrome (PMS). However, Sondheimer et al. (31) reported that routine serum hormonal measures in women with PMS during their luteal phase were not useful in differentiating between patients with PMS and those without PMS. These measures included peripheral luteal phase levels of prolactin, T_4, TSH, and the androgen dehydroepiandrosterone sulfate (DHEAS). These investigators also found the DST not useful in the diagnosis of PMS. The utility of other endocrine challenge tests (e.g., TRHST) in women with PMS is under investigation. The search for hormonal markers for this disorder is an area of continuing study.

Cholecystokinin (CCK) levels have been used in the evaluation of bulimia. Although fasting plasma CCK levels in bulimic patients and nonbulimic controls appear to be equivalent, preliminary research has found that patients with bulimia have blunted CCK peaks compared with controls after eating a standardized liquid meal. Interestingly, some bulimic patients treated with antidepressants show a normalization of CCK responses after eating (as well as an increase in satiety response). This remains a research tool at this time (32).

■ REFERENCES

1. Raj AR, Sheehan DV: Medical evaluation of panic attacks. J Clin Psychiatry 1987; 48:309–313
2. Klee GG, Hay ID: Sensitive thyrotropin assays: analytic and clinical performance criteria. Mayo Clin Proc 1988; 63:1123–1132
3. Orsulak PJ, Crowley G, Schlessor MA, et al: Free triiodothyronine (T_3) and thyroxine (T_4) in a group of unipolar depressed patients and normal subjects. Biol Psychiatry 1985; 20:1047–1054
4. Shader RI, Greenblatt DJ: Thyroid function monitoring for lithium-

treated patients. J Clin Psychopharmacol 1988; 8:81

5. Baker JR, Saunder NB, Wartofsky L, et al: Seronegative Hashimoto thyroiditis with thyroid autoantibody production localized to the thyroid. Ann Intern Med 1988; 108:26–30

6. Gold MS, Herridge P, Hapworth WE: Depression and "symptomless" autoimmune thyroiditis. Psychiatric Annals 1987; 17:750–757

7. Leroy M, Villeneuve A, Lajeunessa C: Lithium and antithyroid antibodies. Am J Psychiatry 1988; 145:534

8. Loosen PT, Garbutt JC, Prange AJ: Evaluation of the diagnostic utility of the TRH-induced TSH response in psychiatric disorders. Pharmacopsychiatry 1987; 20:90–95

9. Loosen PT, Prange AJ: The serum thyrotropin response to thyrotropin releasing hormone in psychotic patients: a review. Am J Psychiatry 1982; 139:405–416

10. Allen CB, Davis BM, Davis KL: Psychoendocrinology in clinical psychiatry, in American Psychiatric Association Annual Review, vol 6. Edited by Hales RE, Frances AJ. Washington, DC, American Psychiatric Press, 1987

11. Targum SD, Greenberg RD, Harmoin RL, et al: Thyroid hormone and the TRH stimulation test in refractory depression. J Clin Psychiatry 1984; 45:345–346

12. Roy-Bryne PP, Uhde TW, Rubinow DR, et al: Reduced TSH and prolactin response to TRH in patients with panic disorder. Am J Psychiatry 1986; 143:505–507

13. Carroll BJ: Dexamethasone suppression test, in Handbook of Psychiatry Diagnostic Procedures, vol 1. Edited by Hall RECW, Beresford TP. New York, Spectrum Publications, 1984

14. Roy A, Pickar D, Doran A, et al: The corticotropin-releasing hormone stimulation test in chronic schizophrenia. Am J Psychiatry 1986; 143:1393–1397

15. American Psychiatric Association Task Force on the Use of Laboratory Tests in Psychiatry: The dexamethasone suppression test: an overview of its current status in psychiatry. Am J Psychiatry 1987; 144:1253–1262

16. Carroll BJ: Informed use of the dexamethasone suppression test. J Clin Psychiatry 1986; 47(supp 1):10–12

17. Nemeroff CB, Evans DL: Correlation between the dexamethasone suppression test in depressed patients and clinical response. Am J Psychiatry 1984; 141:247–249

18. Arana GW, Reichlin S, Workman R, et al: The dexamethasone suppression index: enhancement of DST diagnostic utility for depression by expressing serum cortisol as a function of serum dexamethasone. Am J Psychiatry 1988; 145:707–711

19. Bernstein JP, Chung SY, Avila KSM: Cortisol suppression index: a

new approach to interpreting the DST in depression. J Clin Psychiatry 1982; 43:476–478

20. Martin DM, Climko RP, Sweeney DR, et al: Salivary cortisol analysis: a convenient, noninvasive and cost-effective approach testing. The Psychiatric Hospital 1987; 18:1

21. Nelson RL: Oral glucose tolerance test: indications and limitations. Mayo Clin Proc 1988; 63:262–269

22. McFarland KF, Barker C, Ferguson SD: Demystifying hypoglycemia: when is it real and how can you tell? Postgrad Med 1987; 82:57–65

23. Boyle JR, Schwartz NS, Shah S, et al: Plasma glucose concentrations at the onset of hypoglycemic symptoms in patients with poorly controlled diabetes and in non diabetes. N Engl J Med 1988; 318:1487–1492

24. Lydiard RB: Desipramine-associated SIADH in an elderly woman: case report. J Clin Psychiatry 1983; 44:153–154

25. Blum A: The possible role of tobacco cigarette smoking in hyponatremia of long-term psychiatric patients. JAMA 1984; 252:2864–2865

26. Zubenko GS, Altesman RI, Cassidy JW, et al: Disturbances of thirst and water homeostasis in patients with affective illness. Am J Psychiatry 1984; 141:436–437

27. Kirch DG, Bigelow LB, Weinberger DR, et al: Polydipsia and chronic hyponatremia in schizophrenic inpatients. J Clin Psychiatry 1985; 46:179–181

28. Kramer DS, Drake ME: Acute psychosis, polydipsia, and syndrome of inappropriate antidiuretic hormone. Am J Med 1983; 75:712–714

29. Whalley LJ, Christir JE, Brown S, et al: Schneider's first-rank symptoms of schizophrenia: an association with increased growth hormone response to apomorphine. Arch Gen Psychiatry 1984; 41:1040–1043

30. Bird J, Harrison G: Examination Notes in Psychiatry. Bristol, England, IOP Publishing Limited, Techno House, 1987

31. Sondheimer SJ, Freeman EW, Schonlop B, et al: Hormonal changes in premenstrual syndrome. Psychosomatics 1985; 26:803–810

32. Geracioti TD, Liddle RA: Impaired cholecystokinin secretion in bulimia nervosa. N Engl J Med 1988; 319:683–688

■ ADDITIONAL READING

Toft AD: Use of sensitive immunoradiometric assay for thyrotropin in clinical practice. Mayo Clin Proc 1988; 63:1035–1042

HEMATOLOGIC MEASURES OF POTENTIAL RELEVANCE TO PSYCHIATRISTS

3

Some of these tests (e.g., complete blood count) are routinely employed in the workup of psychiatric patients. Other hematologic tests (e.g., total iron-binding capacity) are supplemental and hence ordered only as indicated.

■ COMMONLY USED HEMATOLOGIC MEASURES

A *complete blood count* (CBC) is almost always a part of a routine screen. The CBC is sensitive to a wide variety of medical disorders that can cause, exacerbate, or mimic psychiatric conditions. Typical components of a CBC include a white blood cell (WBC) count, a differential blood cell count, a red blood cell (RBC) count, hematocrit, hemoglobin, erythrocyte indices, inspection of the peripheral blood smear, and a platelet count.

The *WBC count* (or leukocyte count) is an important test in the evaluation of 1) infectious diseases (leukocytosis or occasionally leukopenia, depending on the infectious agent, can be seen); 2) leukemia; and 3) leukopenia and agranulocytosis, which can be associated with certain psychotropic medications (e.g., phenothiazines, especially clozapine; carbamazepine). Note that lithium treatment is typically accompanied by a benign mild to moderate elevation (e.g., 11,000 to 17,000/μl) of the WBC. The leukopenia often seen in patients taking carbamazepine can frequently be cancelled out in patients taking both carbamazepine and lithium. Neuroleptic malignant syndrome (NMS) can be associated with a leukocytosis (ranging from 15,000 to 30,000/mm^3) in about 40 percent of cases (1).

A *WBC differential* involves the characterization of the types of WBCs that make up the patient's WBC count. If just a WBC count was included in a patient's routine screen, a follow-up WBC differential is often necessary to further interpret an abnormal WBC count. The WBC differential count might involve a search for a potential "shift to the left," where in the granulocyte series there is a significant number of early neutrophilic precursors (band forms) as compared with segmented neutrophils. This shift to left (i.e., from segmented neutrophils to band forms) often suggests bacterial infection. A shift to the left has also been reported in about 40 percent of NMS cases.

The *RBC count* is useful in the diagnosis of anemia and used in the calculation of RBC indices. Elevated RBC counts can be seen in polycythemia.

Hematocrit (Hct) is an important hematologic measure used in the screening, evaluation, and follow-up of anemia. Note that anemia can be associated with a wide range of mental status changes, including asthenia, depression, and psychosis. According to the World Health Organization, at least one-fifth of the world's population, including 20 percent of women in the United States of childbearing age, has iron-deficiency anemia.

Hemoglobin (Hb) is used in the evaluation and follow-up of anemia. Some laboratory clinicians believe that a whole blood Hb measure is a more accurate and reliable screening test for anemia than an Hct.

RBC, or erythrocyte, indices are important determinations for the evaluation and follow-up of anemia. RBC indices include

1. *Mean corpuscular volume* (MCV). Describes the average volume of an RBC. Commonly elevated in alcoholism.
2. *Mean corpuscular hemoglobin concentration* (MCHC). The grams of hemoglobin per deciliter of RBCs; expressed in SI units, it is grams per liter. Therefore, in present units, a normal value ranges from 33 to 37 g/dl, in SI units from 330 to 370 g/ liter.
3. *Mean corpuscular hemoglobin* (MCH). Describes the average hemoglobin weight of each individual RBC. Expressed in picograms of hemoglobin per RBC.
4. *Red cell distribution width* (RDW). Patients sometimes can present with a combination of microcytic and macrocytic anemias. While calculating the MCV, these two anemias might cancel each other out, giving rise to a normal MCV. A high RDW indicates a wide variation in the width of the RBCs and suggests a combined anemia. This can be important in the

evaluation of the chronic alcoholic patient, who can have both vitamin B_{12} and folate deficiencies and iron deficiency (e.g., from gastrointestinal blood loss).

Further characterization of an abnormal CBC can involve inspection of the peripheral blood smear for possible abnormal features such as 1) atypical lymphocytes, suggesting, for example, infectious mononucleosis; 2) hypersegmented neutrophil nuclei, as can be seen in B_{12} or folate deficiencies; 3) primitive blast forms of WBCs suggestive of acute leukemia; 4) toxic granulations in leukocytes; or 5) RBC abnormalities, including hypochromia (suggesting iron deficiency), macrocytosis (as in megaloblastic anemia), microcytosis, sickle cells, elliptocytes, spherocytes, and Howell-Jolly bodies.

■ OTHER HEMATOLOGIC MEASURES

A *reticulocyte count* provides an estimate of RBC production taking place in the bone marrow. It is typically increased in the context of increased erythropoiesis (e.g., secondary to blood-loss anemia or anemia responding to treatments such as B_{12}, folate, or iron administration). It is typically low in disorders of RBC maturation, such as megaloblastic or iron deficiency anemia before treatment. The reticulocyte count is also low in the anemia of chronic disease.

Vitamin B_{12} is a part of the workup of megaloblastic anemia and dementia. Neuropsychiatric symptoms that can be seen in patients with B_{12} deficiency include psychosis, paranoia, fatigue, agitation, marked personality change, dementia, and delirium. Megaloblastic anemia and neuropsychiatric dysfunction can result from a deficiency of either B_{12} or folate (folic acid); hence, serum folate is typically also measured with serum B_{12}. The clinician should note that behavioral and mental status abnormalities have been reported in patients with low B_{12} and/or folate *who did not have abnormal hematologic indices (i.e., macrocytosis or anemia)*. Additionally, patients with B_{12} deficiency can often be without some of the other laboratory abnormalities typically associated with pernicious anemia (PA). For instance, B_{12}-deficient patients can have normal WBC and platelet counts and normal serum lactate dehydrogenase (LDH) and bilirubin; in fact, such findings are probably typical of patients with B_{12} deficiency without the anemia. Lindenbaum et al. (2) suggested that in patients with equivocal laboratory findings for B_{12} deficiency the demonstration of elevated serum levels of methylmalonic acid or total homocysteine is useful in confirming the presence of B_{12} deficiency.

Schilling test is a test utilized by hematologists and internists in the evaluation of megaloblastic anemia and is useful for confirming a diagnosis of PA or B_{12} deficiency. Lindenbaum et al. (2) reported that B_{12} deficiency with neurologic disorder can still be seen in the face of a normal Schilling test result.

Serum vitamin B_{12} intrinsic factor is useful in confirming a diagnosis of PA. Intrinsic factor (IF) is required for the absorption of vitamin B_{12} from the gut (ileum). Vitamin B_{12} forms a complex with IF before being absorbed. When IF is low, PA is diagnosed.

Serum folate (folic acid), used in the evaluation of patients with megaloblastic anemia, is typically measured in conjunction with serum B_{12} levels. Decreased folate levels have been associated with the use of alcohol, phenytoin, oral contraceptives, and estrogens. Mental status changes have been reported in patients with low serum folate levels and otherwise-normal hematologic indices (i.e., no megaloblastic changes). Note that in patients with pernicious anemia folic acid administration can reverse the hematologic abnormalities, but not the neurologic abnormalities.

Serum iron is used in the evaluation of microcytic anemia. Iron is essential for the normal functioning of hemoglobin. Serum iron is typically decreased in iron deficiency anemia. Serum iron values can be increased in cases of accidental or intentional overdoses with iron or iron-containing oral supplements.

Total iron-binding capacity (TIBC), used in the evaluation of microcytic anemia, measures the amount of iron that would appear in the plasma if all the transferrin (the transport protein for iron) were saturated with iron. TIBC is typically increased in iron deficiency anemia; increased TIBC is also possible in patients with blood loss or hepatitis or those taking oral contraceptives. The TIBC is usually decreased in the anemia of infection or chronic disease.

Serum ferritin is thought by some to be the most sensitive test available for detecting iron deficiency (3). Ferritin is a protein capable of sequestering up to 4,500 molecules of iron for future use. Ferritin is produced in direct proportion to the amount of iron present (stored iron). Low serum ferritin is found in iron-deficiency states. Ferritin levels can be increased in certain inflammatory conditions (e.g., infectious disease, rheumatoid arthritis, systemic lupus erythematosus) and in iron overload disorders (e.g., hemochromatosis).

Miscellaneous tests for iron deficiency anemia that can be used by hematologists in the evaluation of iron deficiency anemia include serum transferrin, transferrin saturation, bone marrow biopsies, and iron absorption and excretion studies.

■ COAGULATION TESTS

Prothrombin time (PT) can be elevated in conditions that involve significant liver damage (e.g., hepatitis or cirrhosis). PT is a useful measure of liver function and is often included as a liver function test along with liver enzymes, serum total protein, serum albumin, and serum bilirubin. PT is also used to monitor anticoagulant therapy.

Partial thromboplastin time (PTT) is used to monitor anticoagulant therapy (with heparin). A modification of the PTT is the activated partial thromboplastin time (APTT). The APTT is more sensitive than the PTT and is now more frequently performed than the PTT.

A *platelet count* can be substantially decreased by certain psychotropic medications (e.g., carbamazepine, clozapine, phenothiazines). Many nonpsychotropic drugs can also decrease the platelet count. The platelet count might be decreased alone (i.e., thrombocytopenia) or with all the other blood cell lines (i.e., pancytopenia). Medical conditions in which the platelet count can be reduced include idiopathic thrombocytopenic purpura, leukemias, metastases to the bone marrow, and systemic lupus erythematosus.

■ REFERENCES

1. Janicak PG, Bresnaham DB, Comaty JE: The neuroleptic malignant syndrome: a clinical update. Psychiatric Annals 1987; 17:551–555
2. Lindenbaum J, Healton EB, Savage DG, et al: Neuropsychiatric disor-

ders caused by cobalamin deficiency in the absence of anemia or macrocytosis. N Engl J Med 1988; 318:1720–1728

3. Tilkian SM, Conover MB, Tilkian AG: Clinical Implications of Laboratory Tests, 4th ed. St Louis, MO, CV Mosby Co, 1987

4 BIOCHEMICAL EVALUATIONS IN PSYCHIATRY

■ SERUM ELECTROLYTES

If serum electrolytes (e.g., sodium, potassium, chloride, bicarbonate) have not been ordered as a part of a routine screening battery for a psychiatric patient (as they often are), the psychiatrist is advised to have a fairly low threshold for ordering these tests as part of an augmented evaluation of the patient. Indeed, many neuropsychiatric complications can arise in the patient with electrolyte abnormalities.

SERUM SODIUM

Hyponatremia can be associated with significant mental status changes. Hyponatremia can be seen in some medical and psychiatric disorders, including Addison's disease, the syndrome of inappropriate secretion of antidiuretic hormone (SIADH), and psychogenic polydipsia (compulsive water drinking). The use of carbamazepine has also been associated with hyponatremia (1).

SERUM POTASSIUM

Serum potassium, like sodium, is important in nervous and muscle tissue functioning. Hypokalemia can be associated with significant weakness, fatigue, electrocardiogram (ECG) changes (i.e., flattening of T waves, S-T depression, the appearance of U waves, and cardiac arrhythmias), paralytic ileus, and muscle paresis. Hypokalemia is common in bulimic patients with binge-purge behavior and in psychogenic vomiting. Laxative abuse in binge-purge patients can contribute to hypokalemia. Hypokalemia can also be associated with either diuretic use or abuse. When severe, hypokalemia can be life threatening.

Hyperkalemia can be associated with complications of various medical conditions (e.g., renal failure, Addison's disease). Hyperkalemia can also be seen in overdoses of oral potassium supplements. ECG changes associated with hyperkalemia include peaked T waves, S-T depression, and prolonged P-R intervals and QRS complexes.

SERUM CHLORIDE

Serum chloride, the most abundant extracellular anion, exerts an important influence on acid-base balance. Serum chloride can increase to compensate for decreases in serum bicarbonate. Chloride levels can be decreased in bulimics with binge-purge behavior and in patients with psychogenic vomiting.

SERUM BICARBONATE

Some laboratories substitute the serum bicarbonate with the closely related value of total serum carbon dioxide (CO_2T) or carbon dioxide (CO_2) content. The CO_2T measures the combined concentrations of bicarbonate, carbamino CO_2, carbonic acid, and dissolved CO_2 in blood. Both the bicarbonate and CO_2T are useful in the evaluation of acid-base abnormalities.

Serum bicarbonate has been noted to tend toward lower levels in some patients with hyperventilation syndrome (HVS) and panic disorder. There is often an accompanying mild compensatory elevation in the serum chloride. Bicarbonate might be elevated in patients with bulimia and uncontrolled binge eating and purging, in patients abusing laxatives, and in patients with psychogenic vomiting.

■ RENAL FUNCTION TESTS

Blood urea nitrogen (BUN) increases can be associated with various mental status changes (e.g., lethargy, delirium). Additionally, elevations of the BUN can signal an increased potential for toxicity with some commonly used psychiatric medications, specifically lithium and amantadine, both of which typically experience faulty clearance through the kidneys in the face of BUN elevations. BUN elevations are also seen in dehydrated patients.

Serum creatinine, along with the BUN, is a useful test in the evaluation of renal function. Serum creatinine levels do not become elevated until approximately 50 percent or more of the nephrons of the kidney are damaged. Hence, creatinine determinations are not the most sensitive indicator of early renal disease.

The *creatinine clearance test* is one of the most sensitive evaluations of kidney function. This test is frequently used by psychiatrists in the pretreatment and follow-up laboratory evaluation for the patient treated with lithium, especially in the patient with a history of kidney disease. The creatinine clearance usually is determined by obtaining a 24-hour urine sample, with a serum or plasma creatinine drawn at some point (typically midpoint) during the urine collection period. Although shorter urine collection times are sometimes used (e.g., six- or 12-hour collections), a 24-hour sample is felt to provide the most accurate reflection of creatinine clearance. Generally, the patient needs to be adequately hydrated before the urine collection so that the urine will flow at an average of at least 2 ml/min. Patients are generally told to avoid tea, coffee, and vigorous exercise during the test. Different formulas to calculate the creatinine clearance exist, some using conventional units, others using SI units. One formula using SI units is

Creatinine clearance corrected for body surface area =

$$\frac{\mu mol/liter \text{ (urine creatinine)}}{\mu mol/liter \text{ (serum creatinine)}} \times \frac{\text{total urine volume (ml)}}{s} \times \frac{1.73 \text{ m}^2}{A}$$

where "s" is the time in seconds (in 24 hours there are 1,440 minutes or 86,400 seconds) and "A" is the body surface area in square meters (m²). Nomograms are available for the determination of body surface area using the patient's weight and height. Some laboratories will calculate the creatinine clearance and will correct for body surface area by obtaining the patient's weight and height. Some laboratories will provide the clinician only with urine and serum creatinine values and the measured total urine volume. If the patient is an adult who weighs about 150 pounds, his or her body surface area is 1.73 m^2, and an adjustment for body size is not needed. If only a plasma creatinine concentration is available, formulas to estimate the creatinine clearance are available (2).

Serum and urine creatinine should not be confused with serum and urine creatine. Creatine determination has been used as a measure of muscle damage in various conditions, but now has been largely replaced by creatine phosphokinase (CPK) determinations.

The *24-hour urine protein test* is relevant to psychiatrists because lithium has been reported to cause "nephrotic range" proteinuria (i.e., greater than 3.5 g) in certain patients. Such patients should be carefully evaluated.

Routine urinalysis is important in the detection of a number of disease states of potential significance to psychiatrists. If the psychiatrist has not ordered this as part of a routine screening battery, he or she should have a fairly low threshold for ordering a urinalysis as part of an augmented evaluation, especially in a patient suspected of having urologic disease. A urinalysis can be helpful in detecting and assessing a number of medical conditions (not just related to urologic problems), including diabetes mellitus, diabetes insipidus, SIADH, and hepatobiliary disease. An abnormal urinalysis can provide important clues to the etiology of certain organic mental disorders secondary to certain urologic and systemic disorders.

A routine urinalysis typically includes an evaluation of the urine for

1. *General appearance.* Pink or red-tinged urine can be seen if blood, hemoglobin, or myoglobin is in the urine. It also can be seen in patients who have recently ingested beets or certain food colorings, as well as in patients with porphyria. Urine that turns a bright burgundy after exposure to several hours of bright light is also suggestive of porphyria. Urine that is cloudy and malodorous is suggestive of urinary tract infections.
2. *Urine pH.* For example, an acidic pH can be seen in

ketoacidosis secondary to either uncontrolled diabetes or starvation.

3. *Urine specific gravity*. This provides a quick and easy assessment of the concentrating and diluting ability of the kidneys. The specific gravity of urine might be high in SIADH, diabetes mellitus, or in volume-depletion states. Specific gravity can be low in diabetes insipidus (e.g., secondary to lithium) or excessive water load with normal renal function (e.g., psychogenic polydipsia).

4. *Urine bilirubin*. The presence of bilirubin in the urine is suggestive of biliary tract obstruction.

5. *Urine glucose*. Glucose can be seen in the urine in patients with diabetes mellitus. A false positive is possible in patients who have recently ingested vitamin C.

Also commonly included in a routine urinalysis are tests for blood, ketones, protein, urobilinogen, and nitrites in the urine. Urine sediment analysis—to determine the presence of red blood cells (RBCs), white blood cells (WBCs), epithelial cells, crystals, yeast, parasites, and casts—may also be done. Note that prepackaged and prepared dipsticks (which provide results after briefly placing the dipstick in the patient's urine) can be used to facilitate a quick and easy evaluation of many of these urine determinations (e.g., urine pH, protein, glucose, ketones, bilirubin, urobilinogen, WBCs, hemoglobin, and nitrites). A urinalysis with a dipstick positive for blood and with no RBCs seen on microscopy suggests myoglobinuria. This should be followed up with a urine myoglobin test. This is an important part of a workup for rhabdomyolysis, which can be seen in the context of suicide attempts, illicit drug use (e.g., cocaine, phencyclidine, heroin), straightjacket use, and adverse reactions to antipsychotics (e.g., neuroleptic malignant syndrome). In rhabdomyolysis, other laboratory changes include elevations of serum muscle enzymes—such as creatine phosphokinase (CPK), aldolase, lactate dehydrogenase (LDH), and aspartate aminotransferase (AST)—as well as possible laboratory abnormalities suggesting impaired renal function (serum creatinine, BUN). On a final note, dipstick tests for protein do not reliably detect Bence Jones proteins seen in many patients with certain gammopathies and amyloidosis—disorders that can have neuropsychiatric complications.

To measure *urine sodium*, urine is typically collected from a patient over a 24-hour period. Urine sodium can be elevated 1) in patients treated with lithium, 2) in patients undergoing diuretics therapy, 3) in patients with SIADH, and 4) during postmenstrual diuresis (physiologic). Urine sodium can be low in patients on steroids, in disease states associated with reduced glomerular filtration (e.g., congestive heart failure), and in premenstrual sodium and water retention.

■ OTHER COMMON BIOCHEMICAL TESTS

Other common tests that are often a part of a routine or augmented laboratory evaluation of the psychiatric patient are described below.

Serum calcium is frequently part of a routine blood chemistry screen of a psychiatric patient. This is because abnormalities of calcium metabolism can be associated with a wide range of mental status changes. Hypercalcemia can be associated with weakness, depression, asthenia, and psychosis; ECG changes can include arrhythmias and a shortened QT interval. Hypocalcemia can be associated with depression, irritability, delirium, Chvostek's and/or Trousseau's sign, and tetany, including carpopedal spasm and laryngospasm. Hypocalcemia secondary to hypoparathyroidism should be suspected in patients with a past history of thyroid or parathyroid surgery. Chronic laxative abuse can be associated with hypocalcemia. Hypercalcemia can be seen in cancers involving bone, in vitamin D intoxication, and in conditions associated with excess secretion of parathyroid-like hormones.

Because of the close relationship between calcium and *phosphorus* metabolism, calcium and phosphorus determinations are typically ordered together. Serum parathyroid hormone (PTH) can further assist in the evaluation of serum calcium and phosphorus abnormalities. Phosphorus elevations can be found in hypoparathyroidism or hypervitaminosis D (e.g., in a patient who overzealously takes vitamin D supplements). Serum phosphorus decreases can be found in hyperparathyroidism and celiac sprue. Low phosphate levels have also been associated with HVS and hyperventilation that accompanies a panic attack (3). Gorman et al. (4) reported that inorganic phosphate blood levels tend to be lower in patients with panic disorder than in normal controls (but not necessarily in an abnormal range).

Serum magnesium is commonly decreased in alcoholism. Hypomagnesemia can be associated with significant mental status changes, including agitation and delirium, potentially progressing to convulsions and coma. It can be associated with a positive Chvostek's sign and tetany. Hypomagnesemia is generally an indication for appropriate magnesium replacement.

Total protein is made up of albumin and globulins (e.g., proteins and enzymes, transport proteins, immunoglobulins, and complement). Many of these proteins are responsible for transporting certain psychotropic medications through the bloodstream because most psychotropic agents (e.g., tricyclic antidepressants, antipsychotics, anticonvulsants) are highly protein bound. Hence, low serum protein can result in greater patient sensitivity to conventional doses of these drugs. Lithium is not protein bound.

Total protein can be elevated in severe dehydration or in some of the gammopathies. It can be low in malnutrition, protein-losing gastroenteropathies, and nephrotic syndrome. *Serum protein electrophoresis and immunoelectrophoresis* can characterize protein abnormalities and can be used in the workup of multiple myeloma and other gammopathies—disorders that can be associated with neuropsychiatric complications. These techniques can also be carried out on urine and cerebrospinal fluid.

Total protein and serum albumin can be used in the evaluation of a patient's nutritional status (i.e., protein intake). For instance, these levels would typically be low in severe anorexia nervosa or in severe depression associated with substantial weight loss. Serum albumin can be measured separately from total protein; it also can be low in severe malnutrition, intestinal malabsorption, or liver disease. These two measures of serum protein are useful in the evaluation of liver dysfunction. Indeed, low total protein and albumin levels in a patient with elevated liver enzymes can reflect that the hepatic insult is greater than when just the liver enzymes are elevated and the protein status is normal. Serum total protein and albumin levels are useful in the evaluation of alcoholic liver disease.

Serum bilirubin is used in the evaluation of liver disease and jaundice, both of which can be associated with the use of certain psychotropic agents (e.g., phenothiazines) or with heavy alcohol abuse. Measurements of indirect bilirubin (unconjugated, prehepatic) versus direct bilirubin (conjugated, posthepatic) are often helpful in determining the cause of the bilirubin elevation (e.g., systemic hemolysis versus common bile duct obstruction).

Blood ammonia nitrogen (NH_3), or plasma ammonia, is part of an evaluation for hepatic encephalopathy. Elevations of plasma NH_3 are strongly associated with aberrant mental status changes (i.e., delirium). Asterixis commonly accompanies hepatic encephalopathy. Significant plasma NH_3 elevations can be seen in hepatic failure secondary to severe hepatic disease (e.g., cirrhosis, Reye's syndrome). Blood samples for this test need to be transported to the laboratory on ice.

Urine myoglobulin is used in the evaluation of patients with suspected rhabdomyolysis. Significant urine myoglobulin elevations can be seen in patients whose suicide attempts involved severe electrical shock or muscle crush injury; in patients with neuroleptic malignant syndrome; in patients intoxicated with phencyclidine, cocaine, or D-lysergic acid diethylamide (LSD); and in patients who are in restraints. Myoglobulinuria can result in renal failure. Appropriate medical interventions need to be made in the context of myoglobinuria. Elevations of serum muscle enzymes are also seen.

Urine 5-hydroxyindoleacetic acid (5-HIAA) excretion is increased in patients with carcinoid syndrome. Psychiatric presentations of this syndrome can include depression, hypomania, anxiety, or confusion.

■ ACUTE INTERMITTENT PORPHYRIA

It is important for the psychiatric clinician to be knowledgeable about acute intermittent porphyria (AIP), a condition potentially associated with significant psychopathology, including psychosis and depression. The clinician also needs to be aware that some of the classic features of the syndrome (i.e., episodic abdominal pain, autonomic dysfunction, and neuropathy) are *not* always present or prominent in patients with AIP (5). Tishler et al. (5) stated that "the classic manifestations of intermittent acute porphyria may represent only one facet of this syndrome; these signs and symptoms, while dramatic and life-threatening, may have created a bias in our understanding of this disease." They also reported that the majority of the subjects in their study who had AIP had little in the way of neurologic abnormalities, except for some signs of neuropsychological impairment. Psychiatrically, the patients typically presented with periods of agitated psychosis, apathy, or depression.

LABORATORY EVALUATION

The laboratory diagnosis of AIP is usually made on the basis of elevated urine levels of porphobilinogen (PBG) and δ-aminolevulinic acid (ALA). Note that patients do not necessarily excrete excess amounts of these substances during asymptomatic periods; sometimes elevations of only one of these compounds is seen. Most commercial laboratories have the capability of carrying out these determinations.

PBG can be measured either in a fresh random urine sample for a qualitative determination (e.g., Watson-Schwartz or Hoesch test) or quantitatively from a 24-hour urine collection in a special dark bottle (to prevent light from interacting with the PBG and interfering with the results). A positive Watson-Schwartz or Hoesch determination would typically be followed up by a quantitative 24-hour evaluation. Clinicians who suspect AIP in a patient should collect a 24-hour urine sample for a quantitative measurement whenever possible. *Uroporphyrin* is also commonly elevated during manifest AIP, but less so during asymptomatic (latent) periods.

ALA, in the workup of AIP, is measured in the urine collected over a 24-hour period. Note that ALA can also be elevated in other porphyria syndromes and lead poisoning.

AIP evaluation can include a test to detect diminished activity of *erythrocyte uroporphyrinogen-1-synthetase*. In AIP there is a decrease in this enzyme, which is involved in converting PBG to uroporphyrinogen. Blood samples are required for this test (5).

■ WILSON'S DISEASE (HEPATOLENTICULAR DEGENERATION)

Wilson's disease is an autosomal-recessive condition resulting in an abnormality in metabolism of copper. The disease is characterized by decreased intellectual functioning and the presence of a movement disorder. There can also be accompanying personality changes and psychosis. The onset of the disorder is typically between the ages of 10 and 30. Although the disorder is rare (1/100,000), the physician needs to consider Wilson's disease in the differential diagnosis of a psychotic young adult with a movement disorder.

LABORATORY EVALUATION

Serum ceruloplasmin is a protein involved in the transport and metabolism of copper. The results from this test are low in Wilson's disease, reflecting the decreased hepatic synthesis of this protein. Ceruloplasmin can also be measured in the urine.

Serum copper is low in Wilson's disease.

Urine copper is useful in the diagnosis of Wilson's disease. Urinary copper, measured in urine collected for 24 hours in a metal-free container, is elevated in patients with Wilson's disease.

Other diagnostic tests that might be utilized in the evaluation of Wilson's disease include tissue biopsies of the liver or kidney in search of increased copper deposition.

■ ENZYMOLOGY OF POTENTIAL RELEVANCE TO PSYCHIATRISTS

Amylase (serum) is commonly used in the evaluation of pancreatic disorders such as acute pancreatitis. However, the specificity of this test is limited by the fact that amylase is also secreted by the parotid glands, the gut, and the female reproductive system. Hence, serum amylase elevations can be seen in mumps and other salivary gland diseases, small bowel obstructions, mesenteric thrombosis, pelvic inflammatory disease, or tubal pregnancies (i.e., with rupture). Serum amylase determinations utilized in the evaluation of pancreatic disease are frequently accompanied by measures of *serum lipase*. Lipase is secreted specifically by the pancreas and aids in the interpretation of serum amylase values.

Serum amylase determination has also been proposed as a method to help monitor certain behaviors in bulimic patients, who can be unreliable in their reporting of binge-purge activity. Baseline serum amylase levels of severe binge eaters are reportedly higher than in normal controls or nonbulimic anorexics. The serum amylase level tends to increase after binge-purge activity and declines as bulimic patients stop binge eating and purging. The source of the amylase elevation is probably salivary. Isoamylase determinations might be useful in helping to differentiate between salivary or pancreatic involvement. Pancreatic involvement would also be associated with lipase elevations. It is also important to monitor serum electrolytes in bulimic patients. Low serum potassium and chloride levels, as well as high bicarbonate levels, tend to correspond with periods of uncontrolled binge eating and purging. Abnormal electrolyte values can also help confirm a high amylase value as being supportive of severe binge eating and purging.

Acid phosphatase is commonly used in the evaluation and follow-up (i.e., monitoring treatment response) of patients with carcinoma of the prostate. It can also be elevated in conditions such as benign prostatic hypertrophy, in disorders involving excessive platelet destruction (e.g., idiopathic thrombocytopenic purpura), and in bone disease (e.g., Paget's disease, metastatic cancer to bone).

Alanine aminotransferase (ALT) was formerly referred to as serum glutamic-pyruvic transaminase (SGPT). ALT is especially useful in evaluating and following viral and drug-induced hepatitides. The ratio of ALT to aspartate aminotransferase (AST) is sometimes advocated as being useful in the differential diagnosis of certain liver diseases. In viral and drug-induced hepatitides, ALT elevations commonly exceed AST values.

Aldolase (ALD) is an enzyme found in various tissues (e.g., liver, muscle, pancreas, lung, genitourinary system, blood cells). Therefore, elevations of this enzyme typically do not provide the physician with much specific diagnostic information. It has been reported that 60 to 80 percent of acutely psychotic and schizophrenic patients can have ALD elevations. ALD can be used in the evaluation and follow-up of certain muscle disorders (e.g., Duchenne muscular dystrophy, McArdle's disease, muscle trauma, idiopathic inflammatory myopathy). Assays of other enzymes found in muscle (e.g., AST, LDH, CPK) are useful in the evaluation of muscle disease. Elevations of these muscle enzymes can be caused by intramuscular injections. Patients who abuse ipecac preparations (e.g., certain bulimic patients) can develop a myopathy; serum muscle enzyme levels can be elevated.

Alkaline phosphatase is often used in the evaluation of hepatobiliary disease. Alkaline phosphatase activity can be increased by certain psychotropic medications such as the phenothiazines. Elevations in alkaline phosphatase can reflect a wide range of pathology (e.g., liver disease, bone disease, renal disease, hyperthyroidism, infectious mononucleosis, sarcoid, hyperparathyroidism). Alkaline phosphatase isoenzymes are available to help determine the source of the alkaline phosphatase elevations (e.g., bone isoenzyme, liver I and II isoenzymes, and biliary alkaline phosphatase).

Aspartate aminotransferase (AST) was formerly referred to as serum glutamic-oxaloacetic transaminase (SGOT). AST is commonly used to follow the progress of patients with liver disease and myocardial infarction (MI). AST elevations can be found in many medical conditions, including disorders resulting in damage to the heart, liver, skeletal muscle, lungs, or kidneys; hence, AST has limited specificity. In alcoholic hepatitis, AST is typically thought to be more elevated than ALT. In viral and drug-induced hepatitides, the opposite is generally the case. Note, however, that these rules do not always apply.

Serum creatine phosphokinase (CPK), used in the evaluation of muscle injury, is also used to evaluate and follow patients with neuroleptic malignant syndrome (NMS). Total CPK is reportedly elevated in up to 50 percent of NMS patients. CPK elevations in NMS can range from 2,000 to 15,000 U/liter; elevations over 100,000 U/liter, however, have been reported. Note that intramuscular injections (e.g., from intramuscular antipsychotic medications) can also dramatically increase CPK levels. Rhabdomyolysis has been associated with various forms of substance abuse (e.g., cocaine, phencyclidine, heroin, amphetamines, ethanol, gasoline sniffing). CPK elevations can also occur in patients in restraints and in those experiencing dystonic reactions secondary to antipsychotics. Cases of asymptomatic CPK elevations presumably related to neuroleptic treatment have been reported, although CPK elevations in psychotic patients not on antipsychotics have also been seen.

The isoenzyme CPK-MB is found largely in heart muscle and is important in the evaluation of patients with suspected MI or in the follow-up of patients after an MI. CPK-MB is the enzyme that typically rises the most rapidly and dramatically in patients who have had an MI.

Serum gamma-glutamyl transaminase (GGT) is useful in the detection and follow-up evaluation of many hepatobiliary diseases as well as in the laboratory evaluation of alcoholism, in which GGT is elevated. This test is reportedly useful in the follow-up of alcoholic liver disease and cirrhosis (e.g., to follow progression). The GGT is reportedly elevated in 90 percent of patients with liver disease (6).

Lactate dehydrogenase (LDH) is found in many body tissues and hence can be elevated in a number of medical conditions, including liver disease, MI, megaloblastic anemia (e.g., pernicious anemia), renal disease, and musculoskeletal diseases. Factitious elevations can occur secondary to RBC hemolysis related to improper or rough handling of the blood specimen tube. LDH normally has five isoenzyme variations: LDH_1, LDH_2, LDH_3, LDH_4, and LDH_5.

Serum glutamic-pyruvic transaminase (SGPT) is now increasingly referred to as alanine aminotransferase (ALT). However, many laboratories and clinicians continue to refer to this enzyme by the SGPT designation. For discussion of this enzyme, see alanine aminotransferase (above).

Serum glutamic-oxaloacetic transaminase (SGOT) is now increasingly referred to as aspartate aminotransferase (AST). However, many laboratories and clinicians continue to refer to this enzyme by the SGOT designation. For discussion of this enzyme, see aspartate aminotransferase (above).

LIVER ENZYMES IN ALCOHOLIC PATIENTS

Heavy alcohol intake has been associated with elevations in GGT, ALT (SGPT), and AST (SGOT). In patients who had completed alcoholism treatment, Irwin et al. (7) reported that patients who had resumed drinking were more likely to show increases from baseline in GGT (≥ 20 percent increase), AST (≥ 40 percent), or ALT (≥ 20 percent), compared with abstainers, whose values at follow-up either stayed the same or fell. It should be noted, however, that in severe alcoholic liver disease, resumption of alcohol use might not result in these liver enzyme elevations, due to already severe liver destruction.

■ REFERENCES

1. Yassa R, Iskandar H, Nastase C, et al: Carbamazepine and hyponatremia in patients with affective disorder. Am J Psychiatry 1988; 145:339–342
2. Cockcroft D, Gault MK: Prediction of creatinine clearance from serum creatinine. Nephron 1976; 16:31–41
3. Griez E, Pols H: Blood gas changes and hypophosphatemia in lactate-induced panic. Arch Gen Psychiatry 1988; 45:96
4. Gorman JM, Cohen BS, Liebowitz MR, et al: Blood gas changes and hypophosphatemia in lactate-induced panic. Arch Gen Psychiatry 1986; 43:1067–1071
5. Tishler PV, Woodward B, O'Connor J, et al: High prevalence of intermittent acute porphyria in a psychiatric patient population. Am J Psychiatry 1985; 142:1430–1436
6. Tietz NW, Finley PR: Clinical Guide to Laboratory Tests. Philadelphia, WB Saunders Co, 1987
7. Irwin M, Baird S, Smith TL, et al: Use of laboratory tests to monitor heavy drinking by alcoholic men discharged from a treatment program. Am J Psychiatry 1988; 145:595–599

IMMUNOLOGIC TESTS OF POTENTIAL RELEVANCE TO PSYCHIATRISTS 5

■ INFECTIOUS AGENTS

The *Venereal Disease Research Laboratories test (VDRL)* is a screening test for syphilis. The serum VDRL can be either positive or negative in early (primary) syphilis, but is more sensitive in cases of secondary syphilis. The serum test is typically positive about one to three weeks after the appearance of a syphilitic chancre. A reactive serum can also be quantitated. VDRL titers are usually high in secondary syphilis and tend to be lower or even negative in tertiary syphilis. Positive serum VDRLs should be confirmed with a fluorescent treponemal antibody absorption (FTA-ABS) test. VDRL reactivity decreases after successful treatment for syphilis.

The cerebrospinal fluid (CSF) VDRL is currently the serologic test of choice for detecting central nervous system (CNS) syphilis. In patients strongly suspected of having neurosyphilis who have either positive or negative serum VDRLs and a positive serum FTA-ABS, a CSF VDRL is obtained. Other CSF findings in neurosyphilis can include increases in the cell count, total protein, and gamma globulins. Whereas a positive CSF VDRL is virtually diagnostic of neurosyphilis, a negative test does not necessarily rule out CNS syphilis. A negative test should be evaluated in the context of the clinical situation, CSF protein, and white blood cell (WBC) count.

A number of conditions can give rise to false-positive VDRLs—hence the compromised specificity of the VDRL. These conditions include rheumatic diseases, such as systemic lupus erythematosus (SLE) and rheumatoid arthritis, as well as intravenous drug abuse and certain infectious diseases, such as infectious mononucleosis.

The *rapid plasma reagin test (RPR)* is probably now the most common screening test for syphilis (although the VDRL is still the test recommended for CSF). The test can be quantitated if the screening RPR is reactive. As with the VDRL, the RPR can be followed to assess the success of treatment. It is recommended that for the nontreponemal tests (i.e., RPR and VDRL), laboratories should titrate results to a final end point rather than report results as greater than some arbitrary cutoff (e.g., greater than 1:512), as determination of a final end point permits better assessment of response to therapy with repeat serologic testing. Positive RPRs need to be confirmed with an FTA-ABS. False-positive results can occur for reasons similar to those outlined above for the VDRL.

Fluorescent treponemal antibody absorption (FTA-ABS) measures antibodies to *Treponema palladum*, the causative agent of syphilis. The FTA-ABS is used to confirm positive (reactive) VDRLs or RPRs. However, even if the initial VDRL or RPR is negative, a serum FTA-ABS should be performed if neurosyphilis is suspected. False-positive results can occur in patients with SLE. The FTA-ABS is not carried out on CSF specimens. A positive FTA-ABS typically remains positive for life, even with successful treatment.

Antibodies to Borrelia burgdorferi can be found in patients with Lyme disease. The vector for the *B. burgdorferi* is the deer tick; a rash typically develops days or weeks after a bite by an infected tick. A wide variety of neuropsychiatric symptoms have been reported in patients with this disease, including fatigue, headache, dementia-like symptoms, spastic paresis, and ataxia. These symptoms can appear months to years after the rash associated with the tick bite (indeed, the rash might have gone unnoticed). Both serum and CSF antibodies to the spirochete can be examined in patients suspected of having this disease.

Technical improvements in the accuracy of tests for *B. burgdorferi* are currently being made. Even urine screening tests are under development. There can be a delay in the appearance of serum and CSF IgG antibodies to this organism, and these antibodies may continue to be found in the CSF for an indefinite period after treatment. In most cases of early Lyme disease, the serologic tests for the disease are often negative, and a diagnosis of Lyme disease must be made on clinical grounds (1). In patients manifesting psychiatric disturbance as part of their Lyme disease presentation, this usually represents a later stage of Lyme disease, when the serology is typically positive. False-positive results can be seen in patients with other spirochetal diseases (e.g., syphilis), infectious mononucleosis, and autoimmune disorders. It is important that Lyme disease serology be performed and interpreted in the context of the patient's illness and overall presentation. The clinician should be familiar with risk factors for Lyme disease and the characteristic findings in the various clinical stages of the disease (1). Isolation of the organism from patients is difficult, and techniques to do so have not proven practical in studies reported to date (1).

Patients with *brucellosis* can manifest various psychiatric symptoms (e.g., depression, fatigue, anxiety). The complement-fixation test, useful in detecting chronic brucellosis, is often negative in the early stages of the disease. Brucellosis has been described as primarily an occupational disease, largely involving farmers, livestock producers, meat-packing plant employees, and veterinarians (i.e., those who commonly come into contact with domestic animals, the natural reservoir of brucellosis).

■ HUMAN IMMUNODEFICIENCY VIRUS

Patients infected with the human immunodeficiency virus (HIV) have been commonly reported to have CNS involvement, even in the absence of other signs or symptoms of acquired immune deficiency syndrome (AIDS) or AIDS-related complex (ARC). Indeed, HIV-related CNS involvement has been reported even in the context of negative serum tests for HIV antibodies and in patients with normal T lymphocyte profiles. Similar to the past reputation of CNS syphilis (neurosyphilis), AIDS may be the next "great masquerader" for which psychiatric clinicians will need to remain vigilant (2).

Organic mental disorders related to HIV infection include AIDS dementia, organic personality disorder, and organic affective disorder; psychiatric presentations include chronic mild depression, acute psychosis, and mania (3,4). The neuropsychiatric syndromes can be related to 1) a direct effect of the AIDS virus on the brain and/or 2) other AIDS-related processes adversely affecting CNS functioning (e.g., severe debilitation and nutritional deficiency states, cryptococcal and other meninigitides, meningeal lymphoma, cerebral mass lesions due to infectious agents such as *Toxoplasma gondii* or neoplastic processes like lymphoma or Kaposi's sarcoma).

HIV SYNONYMS

HIV has also been referred to in the literature as lymphadenopathy-associated virus (LAV), human T-cell lymphotropic virus-III (HTLV-III or HTLV-3), and HIV-1. These refer to the same virus. It is this virus that is the causative organism responsible for AIDS. The virus is now most commonly referred to in the literature as HIV. Certain laboratories continue to refer to the virus by its other designations.

HIV TESTS

HIV ANTIBODY TESTS

The two most commonly performed tests for evidence of HIV infection are enzyme-linked immunosorbent assay (ELISA) and the Western blot test. The Western blot test is used as a follow-up confirmatory test for positive results from the ELISA. These tests do not directly measure the HIV itself, but rather antibodies to HIV; hence, these tests are also sometimes referred to as anti-HIV tests. Antibodies to HIV most commonly become detectable between three weeks to three months after exposure to HIV. Other HIV antibody tests as well as antigen tests that are able to detect the presence of the HIV itself are under development. Causes of false-positive ELISA results have included hematologic malignancies, acute deoxyribonucleic acid (DNA) viral infections, and serum reactive for rheumatoid factor (RF) and antinuclear antibodies (ANA). False positives have also been seen in patients with multiple myeloma, primary biliary cirrhosis, primary sclerosing cholangitis, and alcoholic hepatitis. When both ELISA and confirmatory follow-up Western blot are used in laboratories with good quality control, rates of false positives or negatives are extremely low (5).

OTHER TESTS FOR EVIDENCE OF HIV INFECTION

Other tests for HIV infection include the following:

1. *T_4 cell counts.* The T_4 cells are T lymphocytes that are also sometimes referred to as "helper-inducer" cells. The T_4 cells are normally stimulated by antigens to enhance the response of B lymphocytes (which synthesize antibodies). In HIV infection, T_4 counts are depressed (i.e., less than $400/mm^3$).
2. *T_4/T_8 ratio (or T cell "helper-to-suppressor" ratio).* T_8 cells are T lymphocytes that inhibit or suppress B lymphocyte activity. Hence, T_8 cells are sometimes referred to as "suppressor" T cells. In HIV infection, as well as in some other immunodeficiency states, there is a decrease in the T_4/T_8 ratio.
3. *HIV cultures.* The organism can be cultured from infected body fluid or tissue. However, the techniques for HIV culture are currently expensive, time consuming, of low sensitivity, and available primarily at research centers.

TABLE 5-1. **Possible Indications for Human Immunodeficiency Virus (HIV) Testing**

1. Patients who belong to a high-risk group: 1) men who have had sex with another man since 1977; 2) intravenous drug abusers since 1977; 3) hemophiliacs or other patients who have received since 1977 blood or blood product transfusions not screened for HIV; 4) sexual partners of people from any of these groups; 5) sexual partners of people with known HIV exposure—people with cuts, wounds, sores, or needlesticks whose lesions have had direct contact with HIV-infected blood.

2. Patients who request testing. Note that not all patients will admit to the presence of risk factors (e.g., because of shame, fear).

3. Patients with symptoms of AIDS or ARC.

4. Women belonging to a high-risk group who are planning pregnancy or who are pregnant.

5. Blood, semen, or organ donors.

6. Patients with dementia in a high-risk group.

Note. AIDS = acquired immune deficiency syndrome; ARC = AIDS-related complex.

INDICATIONS FOR HIV TESTING

Table 5-1 outlines some important indications for HIV testing. In addition to these indications, the clinician should note that HIV testing is becoming increasingly important in the workup of some patients with dementia (typically in patients who were at conceivable risk for contracting the HIV); this can be particularly relevant in young patients with varying degrees of unexplained dementia. The Centers for Disease Control (CDC) now recognizes HIV-associated dementia as a presentation of AIDS. It is not uncommon for the dementia syndrome to be the sole or primary part of an AIDS symptom picture.

HIV COUNSELING

HIV testing should be performed in conjunction with appropriate pretest and posttest counseling. The physician needs to be sensitive to the potential psychological stress of the patient undergoing HIV testing. Additionally, the physician needs to be aware

TABLE 5-2. **Pretest HIV Counseling**

1. Discuss meaning of a positive result and clarify distortions (e.g., the test detects exposure to the AIDS virus; it is not a test for AIDS).

2. Discuss the meaning of a negative result (e.g., seroconversion requires time, recent high-risk behavior might require follow-up testing).

3. Be available to discuss the patient's fears and concerns (unrealistic fears might require appropriate psychological intervention).

4. Discuss why the test is necessary. (Remember, not all patients will admit to high-risk behaviors.)

5. Explore the patient's potential reactions to a positive result (e.g., "I'll kill myself if I'm positive."). Take appropriate necessary steps to intervene in a potentially catastrophic reaction.

6. Explore past reactions to severe stresses.

7. Discuss the confidentiality issues relevant to the testing situation (e.g., is it an anonymous or nonanonymous setting). Inform the patient of other possible testing options where the counseling and testing can be done completely anonymously (e.g., where the result would not be made a permanent part of a hospital chart). Discuss who might have access to the test results.

8. Discuss with the patient how being seropositive can potentially affect social status (e.g., health and life insurance coverage, employment, housing).

9. Explore high-risk behaviors and recommend risk-reducing interventions.

10. Document discussions in chart.

11. Allow the patient time to ask questions.

Note. HIV = human immunodeficiency virus; AIDS = acquired immune deficiency syndrome.

of the potential psychological impact a positive HIV result might have.

PRETEST HIV COUNSELING

Table 5-2 outlines some of the major points to consider when doing the pretest counseling for a patient about to undergo a test to determine HIV status. It is important to take enough time to do an adequate job with pretest counseling. The counseling session might begin by the clinician discussing with the patient why HIV testing is needed or asking the patient why he or she thinks testing should be done. It is important for the clinician to assess whether the patient's desire for the test is justified or is based on irrational fears. Some patients appear so upset about the possibility of having AIDS that the physician might end up needing to do the test anyway despite no clear history of high-risk behaviors or high-risk blood transfusion. Remember that not all patients will feel comfortable admitting their high-risk behavior.

One of the major purposes of pretest counseling is to lay the groundwork for patients ultimately to receive the results of their HIV test. *Education* about the meaning of the HIV test is important. Hence, clinicians should be knowledgeable about HIV testing and aware of the laws regarding HIV testing that apply to their state or jurisdiction. For instance, in some states there are laws that specifically penalize physicians and other health-care workers who violate patient confidentiality about HIV test results. Additionally, *informed consent* is usually obtained prior to drawing blood for an HIV test. Obtaining informed consent prior to HIV testing is recommended by the CDC; in some localities it is required by law. The informed consent is typically obtained through discussion between the patient and physician, with some discussion about the potential risks (e.g., social discrimination, loss of job) and benefits (e.g., awareness of HIV status and need for follow-up care) of the test. The patient should be aware that anonymous testing centers exist where only the patient would know the test result. The physician should also realize that the medical record is not always confidential. Employers and insurance companies can sometimes gain access to the patient's record. In addition, lawyers can subpoena a medical record; after it is filed in court, the record can become a part of public record. In the situation in which the testing center requires the clinician to inform the patient's sexual partners of positive test results when the patient refuses to do so, the patient should be informed of this possibility during pretest counseling.

The physician should allow the patient time to ask questions. Common questions include "What does a positive HIV test mean?" "Is the test 100 percent reliable?" "Is a negative test a guarantee that I am not infected?" "Will a positive test mean that I have AIDS?" Obviously, to answer these questions the clinician needs to be knowledgeable about the test and the disease or be able to refer the patient to someone more knowledgeable who can more precisely carry out the pretest counseling. Although the patient is often quite anxious and the clinician understandably wants to provide reassurance, the physician should be cautious about being overly optimistic in patients who have clearly engaged in high-risk behaviors. Reassurance should be in the form of providing the patient with clear and meaningful potential plans for action should the result be positive.

POSTTEST HIV COUNSELING

Table 5-3 outlines some of the major issues that should be addressed with a patient who has had HIV testing and is being informed of the result. The physician is advised to document that this discussion has taken place. Patients who are delusional about having AIDS typically find a way to explain away negative testing results and need to have their underlying psychiatric disorder treated.

Physicians are advised to keep abreast of the continually evolving developments in the field of AIDS and HIV testing to be able to make the most informed pretest and posttest counseling comments and recommendations.

■ VIRAL HEPATITIS

Viral hepatitis has been associated with psychiatric symptomatology including depression, asthenia, anxiety, and psychosis. Typically, other physical symptoms accompany the hepatitis, which can vary in presentation from a minor flulike illness to a form of fulminant, fatal liver failure. Liver function tests are elevated, especially alanine aminotransferase (ALT), formerly referred to as serum glutamic-pyruvic transaminase (SGPT).

The major types of viral hepatitis are those caused by the type A or B viruses or the non-A, non-B viruses (one non-A, non-B virus is also now known as the hepatitis C virus). The hepatitis D virus requires the patient to be previously infected with hepatitis

TABLE 5-3. **Posttest HIV Counseling**

1. Interpretation of test result:

   • *Clarify distortion* (e.g., "a negative test still means you could contact the virus at a future time—it does not mean you are immune from AIDS").
   • Ask questions of the patient about his or her understanding and emotional reaction to test result.

2. Recommendations for prevention of transmission (careful discussion of high-risk behaviors and guidelines for prevention of transmission).

3. Recommendations on the follow-up of sexual partners and/or needle contacts.

4. If test is positive, recommendations against donating blood, sperm, or organs and against sharing razors, toothbrushes, or anything else that might have blood on it.

5. Referral for appropriate psychological support:

   • HIV-positive individuals often need to have available a mental health team (assess need for inpatient versus outpatient care; consider individual or group supportive therapy). Common themes include shock of diagnosis, fear of death and social consequences, grief over potential losses, and dashed hope for good news. Also look for depression, hopelessness, anger, frustration, guilt, and obsessional themes.
   • Activate supports available to patient (e.g., family, friends, community services).

Note. HIV = human immunodeficiency virus; AIDS = acquired immune deficiency syndrome.

B virus. It is usually hepatic infection with these agents that is implied by the term *viral* hepatitis. Other less common viral causes of hepatitis include Epstein-Barr virus infection (i.e., as part of infectious mononucleosis), cytomegalovirus (CMV), yellow fever, herpes simplex, ECHO, coxsackie, rubeola, rubella, and varicella. Nonviral infectious causes of hepatitis include tuberculosis, histoplasmosis, toxoplasmosis, syphilis, and borrelia infection. Noninfectious causes of hepatitis include alcohol and drug use.

HEPATITIS B VIRUS

COMMONLY MEASURED HEPATITIS B VIRAL ANTIGENS

Hepatitis B is mainly transmitted through body-fluid contamination (e.g., intravenous drug abuse, sexual contact, needlestick injury, blood or blood product transfusion, tattooing, ear piercing). Hepatitis B virus infection can be evaluated by measuring a number of the virus antigens, including the following:

1. *Hepatitis B surface antigen (HBsAg)*, also known as the hepatitis Australia antigen (HAA), implies active hepatitis B infection when present in serum. It typically disappears during convalescence.
2. *Hepatitis Be antigen (HBeAg)* indicates a greater degree of infectivity, as well as a greater likelihood of progression to chronic liver disease when present in serum beyond 10 to 12 weeks.

DETECTABLE ANTIBODIES TO HEPATITIS B VIRUS

Antibodies to the hepatitis B virus that can be measured in the serum to evaluate infection in a patient include the following:

1. *Anti-HBc IgM* is the IgM antibody to the hepatitis B virus core antigen. Most patients with acute hepatitis B have high titers of this antibody, whereas chronic carriers typically have low or no detectable anti-HBc IgM. It is often considered the best serologic marker of acute hepatitis B, although some patients with chronic hepatitis B continue to demonstrate this antibody.
2. *Anti-HBc total (IgM + IgG)* is the nonimmunoglobulin class-specific assay for anti-HBc. Note that the IgG antibody component can last for a long time, possibly even for life. Patients with acute, chronic, or resolved hepatitis B infections will typically be positive for this assay.
3. *Anti-HBe* is the antibody to the hepatitis Be virus antigen. The presence of this antibody is typically associated with diminishing infectivity.
4. *Anti-HBs* is the antibody to the hepatitis B virus surface

antigen. This antibody typically appears after clinical recovery from the hepatitis, implies immunity, and usually persists for life. It has been recommended that intravenous drug–abusing patients who are not positive for anti-HBs antibody should receive hepatitis B virus vaccination.

Different viral hepatitis antigens and antibodies are detected at the different stages of the illness. Psychiatric symptoms have been reported during all phases of viral hepatitis. On a final note, correlations between HIV and hepatitis B infection as high as 38 percent have been reported.

HEPATITIS A VIRUS

Hepatitis A is mainly transmitted through the fecal-oral route and has been associated with crowding, poor personal hygiene, poor sanitation, food and water contamination, chronic drug use, and close or intimate contact with individuals infected with hepatitis A. Many hepatitis A infections are thought to be subclinical. However, like hepatitis B, there are possible symptoms of hepatitis A infection that can overlap with psychiatric complaints (e.g., asthenia, anorexia, depression). Because the illness is typically less severe and carries a less serious prognosis than hepatitis B, the psychosocial implications of a type A infection are usually less profound. Tests for type A infection include the following:

1. *Hepatitis A viral antigen* (HAAg) can be found in both serum and stool during acute infection.
2. *Anti-HA*, or the antibody to hepatitis A virus, can either be IgM or IgG.
   - *Anti-HA IgM*. This typically appears early in the disease and implies acute or recent infection with hepatitis A virus. It typically disappears within a few weeks of infection.
   - *Total anti-HA (IgG + IgM)*. The IgG antibody follows the development of the anti-HA IgM. The IgG antibody is thought to persist for life and implies past exposure to the hepatitis A virus with immunity.

NON-A, NON-B HEPATITIS

Negative test results for hepatitis A or B might suggest a non-A, non-B hepatitis infection. In the past, a diagnosis of non-A, non-B hepatitis was a diagnosis of exclusion. Recently, a virus thought responsible for much non-A, non-B hepatitis has been identified. Blood tests for this virus are under development and should soon be available (anti-HCV antibody). Risk factors for non-A, non-B hepatitis largely overlap those for hepatitis B. Indeed, there is also evidence that some patients with non-A, non-B hepatitis might have a mutant form of hepatitis B not detectable by current standard laboratory hepatitis B screens (but detectable with research laboratory tests for hepatitis B DNA).

■ EPSTEIN-BARR VIRUS AND CYTOMEGALOVIRUS INFECTIONS

The Epstein-Barr virus (EBV) and cytomegalovirus (CMV) are part of the herpesvirus group. This is a group of viruses that also includes herpes simplex virus type 1 (responsible for cold sores and fever blisters), herpes simplex virus type 2 (the cause of genital herpes), and the herpes zoster varicellosus virus. Diseases associated with these viruses can be due to an acute infection, a latent infection, or a recurrence of illness following a period of latency. Although each of these viruses may be dormant, each seems to occupy a different niche in the body, hence the different clinical presentations with reactivation of each of these viruses. Complications caused by these viruses can be seen in AIDS patients.

The EBV is the causative agent for infectious mononucleosis (IM). In certain patients, infectious mononucleosis has been associated with a wide range of psychiatric symptoms, including asthenia, depression, changes in mental functioning, changes in physical skills and personality, and even psychosis (7). IM is typically a disease of adolescence and is usually associated with asthenia. CMV causes a mononucleosis-like syndrome (e.g., with fatigue, atypical lymphocytes, cervical lymphadenopathy, and sore throat), but usually the patients affected are older. CMV can also reportedly produce a wide spectrum of psychiatric disturbances, including anxiety, confusion, delirium, and affective psychoses (7). In CMV infection, the heterophil antibody tests (e.g., Paul-Bunnell-Davidsohn test and Lee-Davidsohn test), Monospot tests, and EBV-specific antigen and antibody tests, which are positive in IM, are negative in the mononucleosis-like syndromes related to CMV. CMV is probably the most common cause of seronegative mononucleosis. Both EBV and CMV can be involved in infecting the nervous system and causing meningitis, peripheral neuropathy, and Guillain-Barré syndrome.

ACUTE INFECTIOUS MONONUCLEOSIS

The *WBC count* is typically elevated in acute IM (between 10,000 and 20,000/μl), with an increased number of atypical lymphocytes reported in the differential.

Heterophil antibody tests (tests for "heterophil agglutinins for infectious mononucleosis") evaluate for acute IM in patients with symptoms consistent with disease. In IM, heterophil antibody tests might be negative in the context of positive EBV antigen and antibody tests (see below).

The *"Monospot" test* is a simple and convenient slide test for IM-specific antibodies. A positive Monospot test typically correlates with a heterophil antibody titer of greater than 1:28.

EBV-specific antigen and antibody tests are needed because heterophil antibody tests are not specific for EBV disease. EBV-specific tests include the following:

1. Indirect fluorescent antibody (IFA) titers of IgM and IgG against viral capsid antigen (VCA), otherwise known as VCA-IgM and VCA-IgG.   The VCA-IgM is typically elevated in acute-phase serum; VCA-IgG can be found during the acute phase of IM, but VCA-IgG titers can persist long after the clinical illness.
2. IgG against early antigen (EA), which can be divided into the "diffuse" and "restricted" components (EA-D-IgG and EA-R-IgG).   EA antibody suggests relatively recent viremia with EBV.
3. IgG against EBV nuclear antigen, or EBNA-IgG.   Provides further evidence of EBV infection. The EBNA is felt to be a

neutralizing antibody associated with the resolution of acute IM.

Liver enzyme tests—alkaline phosphatase; alanine aminotransferase (ALT), formerly serum glutamic-pyruvic transaminase (SGPT); and aspartate aminotransferase (AST), formerly serum glutamic-oxaloacetic transaminase (SGOT)—are not uncommonly elevated in acute IM. Hyperbilirubinemia can also be seen.

CHRONIC MONONUCLEOSIS-LIKE SYNDROME

For many years now, a chronic mononucleosis-like syndrome has been described (8). No consensus yet exists about whether a chronic mononucleosis-like condition exists as a discrete entity. Some clinicians have described varying degrees of depression and neurasthenia as being associated with chronic mononucleosis. Preliminary evidence suggests that a significant portion of patients complaining of this disorder have underlying psychiatric pathology (although this does not necessarily imply causality). In 1988, a group of physicians and researchers published a working definition of chronic mononucleosis, renaming it chronic fatigue syndrome (9). No consensus yet exists as to what constitutes an adequate evaluation for patients suspected of having this syndrome. What is generally agreed is that patients thought to have a chronic mononucleosis-like fatigue syndrome need to have a careful medical and psychiatric workup to rule out other possible disorders. The relationship of EBV infection to the chronic fatigue syndrome is controversial. Indeed, antibodies to EBV are not found in all patients with the syndrome, and there are associations between the syndrome and other viruses (e.g., CMV, herpes simplex, coxsackie B, and measles virus).

EBV AND DEPRESSION

Various investigators and clinicians have suspected a possible association between EBV and some cases of major depression. Although some studies have claimed to demonstrate a relationship of the virus to some patients with depression, no clear association has yet been demonstrated, and negative studies exist showing no association. However, a few studies have reported high titers of specific serum antibodies against herpes viruses like EBV in some depressed patients (10). Interestingly, transient psychological stress has been reported to cause reversible increases in some of these antibodies (11). However, it is not believed that a routine serologic determination for a possible herpesvirus infection (e.g., EBV, CMV) is necessary in patients with major depression who otherwise do not have signs or symptoms of these viral illnesses (12).

■ SYSTEMIC LUPUS ERYTHEMATOSUS

An autoimmune disorder of relevance to psychiatrists is systemic lupus erythematosus (SLE). The clinical picture of SLE can include psychiatric disturbance (e.g., depression, psychosis, delirium, dementia). Laboratory tests for this disorder include the LE prep and tests for antinuclear antibodies (ANA) and anti-DNA antibodies.

The *LE prep* (i.e., the lupus erythematosus cell preparation) is used in the diagnosis of SLE and in the follow-up of the effectiveness of treatment. Many drugs (e.g., phenothiazines, barbiturates, hydralazine, procainamide, phenytoin) can cause a false-positive result for this test.

Serum antinuclear antibodies (ANA) are found in up to 98 percent of patients with SLE. ANA is also used to monitor treatment for SLE. Although many techniques have been developed to detect ANA, the fluorescent ANA (FANA) continues to be widely used and is thought by many to be the most useful test for screening patients suspected of having a systemic rheumatic disease such as SLE. Different rheumatic diseases have distinct ANA profiles. If the FANA is positive, the immunologic specificity of the ANA is determined. In drug-induced SLE, positive ANA results can be seen in patients taking various drugs (e.g., anticonvulsants, hydralazine, procainamide, phenothiazines) as well as in patients who smoke. DeLisi (13) cited several reports of increased ANA in hospitalized psychiatric patients, even in those patients who had never been treated with neuroleptics (although ANA titers have in the past been correlated with length of antipsychotic treatment). The ANA can be elevated in other connective tissue disorders besides SLE, including mixed connective tissue disease, scleroderma or progressive systemic sclerosis (PSS), and IM.

Anti-DNA antibodies are used in the diagnosis of SLE as well as in following the treatment of the disease. A positive ANA and anti-DNA strongly support the diagnosis of SLE. The anti-DNA test is useful in asymptomatic patients with a positive ANA; a positive anti-DNA in such patients would be strongly suggestive of subclinical SLE. A number of drugs and conditions (see those described for LE prep and ANA test) can cause positive results for anti-DNA antibody tests, although reportedly much less so than for the ANA test. The anti-DNA test has a higher specificity for SLE than the FANA. Indeed, the presence of antibodies to native DNA in abnormal titers is one of the American Rheumatic Association criteria for SLE; the antibody is rarely found in patients with other rheumatic diseases. Unlike ANA titers, increased anti-DNA titers have not been found in schizophrenic patients (13).

Bonfa et al. (14) reported an association between the presence of *anti-ribosomal P protein* and the presence of lupus psychosis. This association, however, does not necessarily imply causality.

Lupus anticoagulant (LA), an antiphospholipid antibody, has been described in some patients taking phenothiazine antipsychotics, especially chlorpromazine (15). LA associated with haloperidol treatment has also been reported. The presence of LA has been associated with a hypercoagulable state, although the patients with LA typically have prolonged partial thromboplastin times (PTTs). These patients commonly also have positive ANAs and false-positive VDRLs. LA is also found in patients with numerous other conditions, including various neoplastic and autoimmune conditions (e.g., SLE), as well as in otherwise-normal individuals.

In addition to the above tests, certain *serum or plasma complement* components (e.g., C3, C4) can be assayed in the evaluation of acute SLE. In patients with acute CNS lupus, plasma levels of complement activation products (C3a and C5a) are typically markedly elevated (16).

■ OTHER IMMUNOLOGIC MEASURES

Erythrocyte sedimentation rate (ESR, or sed rate) is a nonspecific test of infectious, inflammatory, or malignant disease. The ESR is often normal in patients with these diseases and is therefore of limited value in excluding these disorders in patients with vague complaints (17). In the context of an otherwise-normal examination, an increased ESR is usually transitory and seldom reflects serious underlying disease. When there is no immediate explanation for an elevated ESR, it is probably best to repeat the ESR in several months rather than exhaustively search for occult disease (17). The ESR has a place in the diagnosis and management of temporal arteritis and polymyalgia rheumatica (17) and is frequently used in the diagnosis and follow-up of inflammatory disease (e.g., temporal arteritis).

C-reactive protein (CRP), like the ESR, can be used as a nonspecific measure of infection and inflammation (as in autoimmune disease such as rheumatoid arthritis). Increases in the CRP typically precede those of the ESR; decreases of the CRP usually occur before falls in the ESR.

The *direct and the indirect Coombs test* detect autoantibodies against RBCs and are used in the evaluation of acquired immunologic hemolytic anemias (e.g., secondary to SLE—drug-induced or idiopathic). Some drugs associated with hemolytic anemia include chlorpromazine, phenytoin, levodopa, and methyldopa.

Tests for food allergy and hypersensitivity (e.g., radioallergosorbent test, skin tests) have not proven useful in assessing psychiatric symptoms believed to be related to food allergy and hypersensitivity. Psychiatric symptoms secondary to such food sensitivity have not been clearly demonstrated.

■ REFERENCES

1. Duffy J, Mertz LE, Wobig GH, et al: Diagnosing Lyme disease: the contribution of serologic testing. Mayo Clin Proc 1988; 63: 1116–1121
2. Khouri PJ: Cerebral manifestations of HIV infection. Carrier Foundation Letter 1988; 130:1–2
3. Perry S, Jacobs O: Neuropsychiatric manifestations of AIDS-spec-

trum disorders. Hosp Community Psychiatry 1986; 37:135–142

4. Gabel RH, Barnard N, Nork M, et al: AIDS presenting as mania. Compr Psychiatry 1986; 27:251–254

5. Burke DS, Brundage JF, Redfield RR, et al: Measurement of the false positive rate in a screening program for human immunodeficiency virus infections. N Engl J Med 1988; 319:961–964

6. Beckett A, Summegrad P, Manschreck T, et al: Symptomatic HIV infection of the CNS in a patient without clinical evidence of immune deficiency. Am J Psychiatry 1987; 144:1342–1344

7. Hendler N: Infectious mononucleosis and psychiatric disorders, in Viruses, Immunity and Mental Disorders. Edited by Kurstak E, Lipowski ZJ, Morozov PV. New York, Plenum Press, 1987

8. Holmes GP, Kaplan JE, Stewart JA, et al: A cluster of patients with a chronic mononucleosis-like syndrome: is Epstein-Barr virus the cause? JAMA 1987; 257:2297–2302

9. Holmes GP, Kaplan JE, Gantz NM, et al: Chronic fatigue syndrome: a working case definition. Ann Intern Med 1988; 108:387–389

10. Gotlieb-Stematsky T, Zonis J, Arlazoroff A, et al: Antibodies to Epstein-Barr virus, herpes simplex type 1, cytomegalovirus and measles virus in psychiatric patients. Arch Virol 1981; 67:333–339

11. Glaser R, Kiecolt-Glaser JK, Speicher CE, et al: Stress, loneliness and changes in herpes virus latency. J Behav Med 1985; 8:249–260

12. Amsterdam JD, Henle W, Winokur A, et al: Serum antibodies to Epstein-Barr virus in patients with major depressive disorder. Am J Psychiatry 1986; 143:1593–1596

13. DeLisi LE: Immunologic studies of schizophrenic patients, in Viruses, Immunity, and Mental Disorders. Edited by Kurstak E, Lipowski ZJ, Morozov PV. New York, Plenum Press, 1987

14. Bonfa E, Golombeck SJ, Kaufman LD, et al: Association between lupus psychosis and anti-ribosomal P protein antibodies. N Engl J Med 1987; 317:265–271

15. El-Mallakh RS, Donalson JO, Kranzeler HR, et al: Phenothiazine-associated lupus anticoagulant and thrombotic disease. Psychosomatics 1988; 29:109–112

16. Belmont HM, Abramson S: Lupus psychosis and anti-ribosomal P protein antibodies (letter). N Engl J Med 1988; 323–324

17. Sox HL, Liang MH: The erythrocyte sedimentation rate: guidelines for rational use. Ann Intern Med 1986; 104:515–523

6 TOXICOLOGY OF POTENTIAL RELEVANCE TO PSYCHIATRISTS

Prescribed medications, illicit drugs, and environmental toxins can be involved in generating a wide array of psychiatric symptoms. Because exposure cannot always be reliably determined by a patient's history, laboratory confirmation of suspected exposure is useful, although sometimes difficult to obtain. Accurate psychiatric diagnosis necessitates the clinician's careful attention to toxicology issues. In this guide, the word *medication* typically refers to legitimately prescribed medications that are not being abused. The word *drug* generally refers to illicit drugs (i.e., drugs that are being abused, such as marijuana, cocaine, or heroin).

■ MEASUREMENT OF MEDICATION BLOOD LEVELS

A large number of psychotropic and nonpsychotropic medications can be associated with a wide range of adverse psychiatric side effects (e.g., delirium, medication-induced depression, mania, anxiety, psychosis). It is not uncommon for psychiatric patients to be taking some of these medications for concomitant nonpsychiatric medical disorders. Blood levels for many of these medications, especially the cardiac, anticonvulsant, and respiratory medications, can be determined in most commercial and hospital laboratories; meaningful therapeutic and toxic ranges have been established for these medications. Adverse psychiatric sequelae are most common when the medication blood levels are in the toxic range. However, untoward psychiatric reactions to these medications can sometimes be seen even when the blood level is in a so-called therapeutic range. Medically ill and elderly patients seem particularly sensitive to adverse behavioral and cognitive reactions to these medications.

Table 6-1 lists a number of medications for which meaningful blood levels can be obtained. Different laboratories may utilize differing reference ranges. Check with the laboratory that

TABLE 6-1. **Some Nonpsychiatric Medications with Described Blood Levels**[a]

Medication	Blood Level/Present Units (SI Units)
Acetaminophen	
toxic	>5 mg/dl
	(>330 μmol/liter)
Chlorpropamide	
therapeutic	75–250 mg/liter
	(270–900 μmol/liter)
Dicumarol	
therapeutic	8–30 mg/liter
	(25–90 μmol/liter)
Digoxin	
therapeutic	0.5–2.2 ng/ml
	(0.6–2.8 nmol/liter)
toxic	>2.5 ng/ml
	(>3.2 nmol/liter)
Disopyramide	
therapeutic	2.0–6.0 mg/liter
	(6–18 μmol/liter)
Isoniazid	
therapeutic	<2.0 mg/liter
	(<15 μmol/liter)
toxic	>3.0 mg/liter
	(>22 μmol/liter)
Lidocaine	
therapeutic	1.0–5.0 mg/liter
	(4.5–21.5 μmol/liter)
Procainamide	
therapeutic	4.0–8.0 mg/liter
	(17–34 μmol/liter)
toxic	>12.0 mg/liter
	(>50 μmol/liter)
Propranolol (Inderal)	
therapeutic	50–200 ng/ml
	(190–770 nmol/liter)
Quinidine	
therapeutic	1.5–3.0 mg/liter
	(4.6–9.2 μmol/liter)
toxic	>6.0 mg/liter
	(>18.5 μmol/liter)

TABLE 6-1. **Some Nonpsychiatric Medications with Described Blood Levels[a] (cont)**

Medication	Blood Level/Present Units (SI Units)
Salicylate	
toxic	>20 mg/dl
	(>1.45 mmol/liter)
Sulfonamides (as sulfanilamide)	
therapeutic	10.0–15.0 mg/dl
	(580–870 μmol/liter)
Theophylline	
therapeutic	10–20 mg/liter
	(55–110 μmol/liter)
Tolbutamide	
therapeutic	50–120 mg/liter
	(180–450 μmol/liter)

Note. Blood levels for other medications are also available (e.g., focainide, mexiletine, amiodarone, metoprolol, verapamil, diltiazem, dantrolene, cimetidine, and many antibiotics). Check with your laboratory. From Young DS: Implementation of SI units for clinical laboratory data: style specifications and conversion tables. Ann Intern Med 1987; 106:114–129.

[a]Check with your laboratory for the therapeutic and toxic blood levels that best apply. Quoted blood levels will vary.

you use for the normal reference ranges. Additionally, more extensive toxicology information is frequently available from local poison control centers. Phone numbers for these centers are usually listed in local phone books or are available through local phone operators.

INDICATIONS FOR A PSYCHIATRIST TO OBTAIN A QUANTITATIVE DETERMINATION OF MEDICATION BLOOD LEVELS

Any patient with a recent onset of mental status changes who is taking any of the medications outlined in Table 6-1 should have the blood medication level determined as part of the initial laboratory evaluation. The measurement of medication blood levels is encouraged because of the frequent close proximity of the therapeutic and toxic ranges. For instance, an anxious patient on theophylline should have a theophylline blood level checked; a patient presenting with hallucinations and delirium on phenytoin should have a phenytoin blood level checked (along with an electroencephalogram). In a patient who might have taken an overdose, qualitative analysis of the gastric contents (if available) is recommended in addition to the blood levels. Indeed, such a qualitative analysis of gastric contents can help direct the ordering of blood levels of previously unsuspected medications (or drugs of abuse).

PSYCHOTROPIC BLOOD LEVELS

Indications for obtaining blood levels of psychiatric medications are covered in Chapter 8. Psychotropic blood levels are also obtained in the context of a psychotropic medication overdose, along with analysis of the gastric contents (if available).

■ SUSPECTED DRUG ABUSE

INDICATIONS FOR ORDERING A DRUG ABUSE SCREEN

It is probably best for the clinician to have a relatively low threshold for ordering drug screens in patients who are at high risk of illicit drug use, especially in the context of a patient presenting with unexplained behavioral symptoms. Indeed, because a patient's history regarding drug use is so often unreliable, some clinicians argue that a drug screen should almost always be a part of a routine screening battery for psychiatric patients, even if the patients are not clearly in the potentially high-risk groups. For instance, even geriatric patients have been reported to use illicit drugs. The clinician should remember that drug-induced psychiatric disorders can frequently mimic a number of psychiatric conditions (e.g., depression, anxiety disorders, psychosis). Additionally, substance-induced organic mental disorders can exacerbate symptoms of an underlying idiopathic psychiatric illness.

Specific indications for ordering a drug abuse screen might include 1) patients with a history of illicit drug use or dependence, 2) patients from high-risk groups (e.g., adolescents, entertainers, patients with criminal records), and 3) patients with unusual or unexplained behavioral symptoms or psychiatric presentations.

Again, the clinician should remember that historical information offered by patients related to their illicit drug use is often unreliable; hence, a decision not to order a drug screen based solely on a patient's negative history can be a mistake.

An additional indication for ordering a drug abuse screen is for the follow-up monitoring of illicit drug use as a part of a treatment plan for the drug-abusing patient. In this context, the drug screen obtained can either be planned or random (i.e., surprise checks). (Some clinicians object to the use of the term *random* because it often implies "arbitrary.") Random checks help to detect drug use between scheduled drug abuse screens and generally make it more difficult for the drug-abusing patient to prepare to "fool" the scheduled drug test. These repeat drug screens in the context of drug abuse treatment can be a measure of the effectiveness of the drug program as well as provide additional motivation to the patient to maintain abstinence. Patients are often relieved rather than offended when urine drug testing is included as part of the treatment plan because it helps patients to resist their drug craving to know that discovery and subsequent negative consequences (e.g., loss of hospital privileges, treatment termination, employer or parole officer notification) are a real possibility.

LABORATORY METHODOLOGIES FOR MEASURING ILLICIT DRUGS

The clinician needs to be aware that different laboratory test methodologies exist for the detection of illicit drug use. These include thin-layer chromatography (TLC), enzyme-multiplied immunoassay technique (EMIT), and gas chromatography–mass spectrometry (GC-MS). Some of the drugs and their metabolites measured by these tests include phencyclidine (PCP), cocaine (and its metabolite benzoylecgonine), tetrahydrocannabinol (THC), methamphetamine (and its metabolite amphetamine, as well as other related amphetamines, such as 3,4-methylene dimethoxy-methamine [MDMA, or "ecstasy"]), morphine (and its metabolite morphine-3-glucuronide), and codeine. Some other drugs of abuse that can be tested for include barbiturates, benzodiazepines, other cannabinoids, methadone, methaqualone, propoxyphene, D-lysergic acid diethylamide (LSD), and alcohol.

Different hospital and commercial laboratories employ different techniques in their drug-screening procedures. Additionally, different "limits of detection" might be chosen among the various laboratories. For instance, some laboratories might call a drug screen positive if the substance can be detected at low or intermediate concentrations; other laboratories might call test results positive only if the drug can be detected at high concentrations. False-positive results tend to increase at the lower levels of detection.

The most commonly used screening test for illicit drugs seems to be EMIT. Other common confirmation test methodologies include TLC and GC-MS (1). Some laboratories use TLC as their primary screen. Detection tests for illicit drugs are available either in the form of broad drug screens, which evaluate for the presence of a number of drugs of abuse, or in the form of an individual test for a specific drug.

TLC is currently enjoying an improved reputation for reliability (e.g., Toxi-lab TLC by Marion). EMIT is currently a widely used screening test. With the EMIT drug screens, false positives tend to increase with lower cutoff values (with a corresponding fall in false negatives). Differences in the lower cutoff values used in different studies might account for some of the variations in the false-positive rates for various drugs reported for EMIT in the literature. EMIT, however, remains a very popular and relatively inexpensive drug abuse screen that is considered reliable when properly used. Radioimmunoassay (RIA) has also been utilized as a drug abuse screen.

GC-MS is perhaps the most sensitive and reliable test for illicit substances, but it is also the most expensive. Using more specific and sensitive measurement techniques such as GC-MS, the number of true positives can be increased and the number of false positives decreased. GC-MS is not available in all laboratories.

DRUG-TESTING STRATEGIES

A preliminary drug screen might utilize a less expensive drug test (e.g., EMIT or TLC). The follow-up tests can be confirmed by a different and hopefully more sensitive test (e.g., GC-MS). However, TLC is a common confirmatory methodology when different methodology was used in the screening process (1).

MEANINGS OF A POSITIVE RESULT

Some laboratories will not report a substance as positive unless the presence of the substance was confirmed by at least one follow-up method (that differed from that used in the initial screening procedure). For certain substances, some laboratories might require a second confirmation (reconfirmation) prior to providing a positive report. However, some laboratories will provide positive reports based on the results of an initial screening procedure alone.

DRUG ABUSE TEST RELIABILITY

Some laboratories using the same or different methodologies to test for illicit drug abuse might be more reliable than others. Drug-screening tests reportedly can have significant numbers of false-positive results. For instance, in certain populations where EMIT was used, false-positive rates as high as 10 percent for cocaine, 12.5 percent for amphetamines, 19 percent for THC, and 5.6 percent for opiates have been described (2). Factors leading to false-positive results include 1) medically prescribed medications that interfere and test positive for an illicit drug when certain methodologies are used, 2) test operator errors, 3) equipment contamination (e.g., from previous positive specimens), 4) sample mislabeling, and 5) lack of or inappropriate follow-up confirmatory testing. Some causes of false-negative test results include 1) specimen tampering due to specimen substitution, diluting urine samples, and applying to the urine samples additives that alter the specimen pH and interfere with the test (e.g., salt, baking soda, bleach, perfumes) and 2) improper specimen handling (e.g., allowing a specimen to stand at too high a temperature), permitting the degradation of the drugs that are to be measured. Careful attention to specimen collection and storage procedures and an unbroken "chain of custody" for the specimen can minimize some of these problems.

It has been claimed by the American Association for Clinical Chemistry (AACC) that the accuracy of tests for abused drugs can reach almost 100 percent in laboratories adhering to proper procedures. Laboratories can increase their reliability by having 1) an external quality control program, 2) a staff of professionally trained personnel and laboratory scientists, and 3) training for continued education and refinement of techniques.

SPECIMENS USED IN DRUG SCREENS

The most commonly used specimen in the analysis of possible recent substance use is urine; however, specimens can include blood, breath, saliva, and (in certain instances) a piece of the patient's hair. Cocaine metabolites are excreted in the urine for longer periods than cocaine can be found in blood; hence, urine screens for cocaine are usually superior to blood sampling. All common drugs of abuse, including alcohol, can be measured in urine samples.

Tests for plasma or serum determinations of a large number of drugs of abuse are available. The use of blood samples can decrease the likelihood of specimen tampering by the patient. The use of two sources for samples (e.g., urine and blood) can allow corroboration of the results from the other source (although this clearly increases expense). In general, blood or urine drug levels do not correlate well with clinical findings, and although they do confirm drug use, the levels themselves are not particularly useful in guiding clinical management. In patients suspected of being intoxicated with alcohol, a blood alcohol level (BAL) can be obtained and is useful in helping to assess tolerance (e.g., higher levels in an awake and conscious individual imply greater tolerance). Although lethal BALs are often cited as being between 300 and 400 mg/dl, some chronic alcoholics have developed significant tolerance and can have BALs approaching or exceeding these levels without fatality. Intoxicating BALs are typically in the range of 100–300 mg/dl. Although patients with pathologic intoxication might have low BALs, a low BAL in a patient who appears quite intoxicated should suggest the possibility of other psychoactive substances affecting the patient's clinical state. A nonalcoholic disinfectant should be used at the time of a blood draw for a BAL. Patients suspected of abusing alcohol for long periods commonly have other laboratory abnormalities—such as elevated liver enzymes, typically serum glutamic-oxaloacetic transaminase (SGOT) greater than serum glutamic-pyruvic transaminase (SGPT); bilirubin elevation; and anemia, typically macrocytic.

Breath analysis is also frequently used to screen for recent alcohol intake. Different types of breath alcohol instruments exist, including 1) chemical reagent tube tests, 2) electrochemical cells that generate a voltage in response to alcohol vapor, and 3) tests that utilize infrared detectors of alcohol. Such breath analysis can be used roadside by police officers for individuals suspected of driving under the influence of alcohol or by psychiatric or alcohol units for patients with a history of alcohol abuse who are suspected of being under the influence.

Saliva tests for marijuana are currently available. Hair analysis for PCP abuse is under investigation (3). Finally, a drug screen that does not require obtaining a body specimen is under development. The device (Veritas® 100 Analyzer) utilizes electronystagmography (ENG) waveforms to detect specific drugs of abuse; waveforms reflecting eye movement are collected through electrodes placed on the sides of the patient's eyes.

■ ENVIRONMENTAL TOXINS

Literally thousands of environmental toxins exist that can contaminate the air we breathe, the water we drink, the food we eat, and the materials we touch. These toxins can be found in and around our homes and work environments. The concentrations of these toxins can be quite high in some localities and work environments. Exposure to a number of these environmental toxins has been associated with various behavioral abnormalities. It is important for the clinician to have an appreciation of some of these toxins and an understanding of some of the mental status changes that can be associated with exposure to them so that when the clinician has a high index of suspicion of environmental toxin exposure, the appropriate laboratory tests can be ordered. The patient's current and past occupational history is vital for evaluating possible environmental toxin exposure. Tables listing a wide variety of occupations with their associated potential toxin(s) exposure are available (4).

HEAVY METAL INTOXICATION

Included in this list of potential environmental behavioral toxins are heavy metals such as lead, mercury, manganese, arsenic, and aluminum. If heavy metal exposure is suspected, a determination of blood or urinary concentrations of these heavy metals might be indicated. If the type of heavy metal exposure is unclear, a urine or blood heavy metal screen, which tests for multiple heavy metals (e.g., arsenic, cadmium, lead, mercury, thallium, manganese), can be obtained. For some of these heavy metals, local poison control centers and state departments of public health can assist in locating laboratories capable of performing the necessary tests. Care must be taken to avoid possible artifactual contamination of the sample (e.g., the urine or blood samples should be collected in metal-free containers).

LEAD POISONING

A patient with lead intoxication (plumbism) can manifest apathy, irritability, anorexia, and confusion (e.g., secondary to lead encephalopathy). In adult lead intoxication, neurasthenic symptoms are the most common (4). Although there is an increased awareness about the dangers of lead poisoning today, there are still large numbers of adults and children who continue to be toxic with elevated "body lead burdens" (5). If capillary blood is drawn from the fingertip of a child in the evaluation of possible lead poisoning, care must be taken to reduce the risk of lead contamination from the skin by properly washing the puncture site. Samples used in the evaluation are commonly either blood or urine. Generally, a 24-hour urine is collected in a lead-free container. A lead mobilization test involving the parenteral administration of calcium disodium edetate ($CaNa_2$ EDTA) followed by a 24-hour urine collection has been described. The ratio of micrograms of lead excreted to milligrams of EDTA given is determined; if this is elevated, the result suggests lead intoxication. The free erythrocyte protoporphyrin (FEP) is considered the best screening test for chronic (but not acute) lead intoxication (4), although both an FEP and a blood lead level should be obtained. An iron deficiency anemia can cause an elevation in the FEP. Elevated red blood cell (RBC) zinc protoporphyrin levels can also reflect increased body lead burdens.

There is no complete consensus at this time as to the lower "threshold" blood lead level that can give rise to detectable neurobehavioral toxicity. Landrigan et al. (5) suggested that "subclinical dysfunction" can be observed at blood lead levels as low as 30 $\mu g/dl$ in adults and 15 $\mu g/dl$ in children. Goldman and Baker (6) suggested the central nervous system "no effect" range to be between 40 and 60 $\mu g/dl$. The Centers for Disease Control has labeled levels greater than 25 $\mu g/dl$ excessive for children.

Other studies used in the laboratory evaluation of lead poisoning include urinary coproporphyrin (UCP) and δ-aminolevulinic acid (ALA).

MERCURY, MANGANESE, ARSENIC, AND ALUMINUM POISONING

Neuropsychiatric symptoms that have been associated with *mercury* intoxication include psychosis, fatigue, headache, apathy, decreased memory, and emotional lability. Contemporary routes of exposure include inhalation or ingestion of inorganic mercury or mercury-containing compounds (e.g., in fungicides). Such exposure can occur in individuals involved in the manufacturing of thermometers, incandescent lights, X-ray machines, mirrors, vacuum pumps, felt hats, and paper and in those involved in the electrochemical industry. Mercury vaporizes at room temperature, making inhalation an easy route of entry into the body. Mercury can also be absorbed through the skin. Mercury can contaminate water and fish supplies if improperly disposed of by certain industries. Laboratory specimens for this heavy metal can include blood, urine (collected in a metal-free container), and even hair. It is felt that the segment of hair positive for mercury accurately reflects the blood mercury level at the time the hair was formed.

Hair analysis and urine and serum *manganese* determinations can be utilized for an evaluation of possible manganese poisoning. Manganese poisoning can be associated with a progressive psychiatric condition known as "manganese madness" and a Parkinson-like syndrome. Individuals can be exposed to substantial amounts of manganese dust during manganese mining operations.

Arsenic poisoning can present with symptoms including extreme fatigue, blackouts, hair loss, hyperkeratosis of the palms and soles, and anemia. Exposure to arsenic can be seen in the home or workplace from arsenic-containing pesticides, rodenticides, and herbicides and from work in the manufacture of brass, bronze, ceramics, dye, and paints. Additionally, burning wood pressure treated with chromated copper arsenate (CCA) can result in arsenic poisoning simply by inhaling the smoke or from skin contact with burned ash. Arsenic can be measured in whole blood, serum, urine, hair, or nails. Because of the short half-life of arsenic in blood, urine is the preferred sample. Urine, hair, and nail specimens can be used for evaluating chronic exposure.

Aluminum can be measured in the serum or the urine. It should be collected in a metal-free container. Increases in serum aluminum can be seen in patients with renal failure secondary to using aluminum-containing antacids or from dialysis machines utilizing a high-aluminum dialysate. High serum aluminum levels have been associated with dialysis dementia. Consequently, aluminum is now routinely removed from the water used in kidney dialysis. Aluminum has also been implicated by some investigators in the etiology of some forms of dementia (e.g., Alzheimer's disease and Guamanian Parkinson-dementia-ALS complex), but work in this area is preliminary and inconclusive.

MISCELLANEOUS TESTS FOR POTENTIALLY CLINICALLY SIGNIFICANT HEAVY METAL EXPOSURE

Serum aminolevulinate dehydratase can be decreased in lead and other types of heavy metal poisoning and can be useful in the detection of subclinical lead poisoning.

Aminolevulinic acid can be measured in urine (typically a 24-hour collection) or serum. Aminolevulinic acid can be elevated in lead poisoning and porphyria (e.g., acute intermittent porphyria).

ORGANIC ENVIRONMENTAL TOXINS AND SOLVENT-INHALANT ABUSE

Exposure to these organic environmental toxins can be related to occupational or residential exposure or to some forms of abuse. Many of these toxins, e.g., insecticides (and repellants), rodenticides, formaldehyde, and organic solvents, have the potential for causing behavioral aberrations. Blood or urine tests to detect most of these organic compounds are not readily available.

State departments of public health can usually be of assistance in performing analyses relating to suspected cases of occupational exposure.

As alluded to earlier, neuropsychiatric syndromes secondary to organic toxins can be seen in the context of intentional exposure (i.e., in abusers or as a part of a suicide attempt). Chronic abusers of leaded gasolines can often be identified by laboratory evidence of lead poisoning (e.g., basophilic stippling of RBCs, increased 24-hour urine lead levels, and increased erythrocyte protoporphyrin levels) (7). Chronic solvent abusers in general might also demonstrate abnormalities in kidney, liver, lung, hematologic, and cardiovascular functioning. Abused solvent-inhalants such as amyl and isobutyl nitrite, Freon®, butane (e.g., from cigarette lighters), or formaldehyde can sometimes be detected in the emergency room by the use of gas chromatographic analysis of a blood specimen. (Consult with your laboratory for details.) Chronic toluene abuse (toluene can be found in glues, paints, lacquers, adhesives, inks, and cleaning fluids) has also been associated with certain magnetic resonance imaging (MRI) abnormalities (e.g., brain atrophy and loss of gray-white matter differentiation).

Acute and chronic exposures to various organic solvents in the workplace (or related to chronic abuse) have been associated with various neuropsychiatric effects including panic attacks (8). Long-term exposure to solvents has been related to organic personality disorders, sometimes variously referred to as "painter's syndrome" or "solvent encephalopathy." Again, suspected organic toxin exposure is typically supported by a thorough history. Laboratory confirmation is often difficult because specialized laboratory equipment and expertise are necessary for the evaluation of possible contamination with many of these substances. Local poison centers may be of assistance in locating laboratories capable of performing analyses for some of these substances.

■ MISCELLANEOUS TOXICOLOGY ISSUES

In the past, *bromide* intoxication (bromism) was a common cause of organic mental disorder because inorganic bromide salts and bromide-containing compounds were frequently used as sedatives, hypnotics, and anticonvulsants. Today, the use of bromide in these sorts of medications is rare; however, some older bromide-containing sedatives are still used by individuals who have stock-piled some of these medications. Bromide intoxication can produce psychosis, hallucinations, delirium, and eventually coma. A serum bromide level can be an important supplementary diagnostic test when some form of bromide ingestion and intoxication is suspected.

Sometimes serum bromide levels are suggested as part of an organic brain syndrome (e.g., dementia workup), especially when serum chloride is elevated. The serum chloride might appear elevated in patients with bromide intoxication because most laboratory methods that measure chloride lack the specificity to adequately differentiate chloride from bromide.

Caffeine blood levels can be measured in serum or plasma. A caffeine blood level can be used in the evaluation of the patient with suspected caffeinism. Patient compliance with recommended caffeine restriction can also be followed by a caffeine blood level. Caffeine plasma levels reportedly peak 45 minutes to two hours after ingestion. The half-life in normal adults is about three to seven-and-a-half hours (4).

Serum vitamin A levels may be elevated in patients who overzealously ingest vitamin A supplements. Hypervitaminosis A can be associated with mental status changes (e.g., depression, asthenia, and delirium). Increased intracranial pressure (pseudo-tumor cerebrei) can also be seen.

Laxative abuse can be seen in certain psychiatric patients (e.g., those with anorexia or bulimia) and in some patients with factitious disorders. Laxative abuse can be the cause of chronic diarrhea in patients who have undergone extensive workups for their diarrhea. Abnormal laboratory findings can include hypo-calcemia and other electrolyte abnormalities. Screening tests to detect laxative abuse in stool or urine specimens have been described (4). The clinician might want to consult with their laboratory to discuss ways to detect surreptitious laxative use in a particular patient.

Anabolic steroid abuse can cause psychiatric complications that range from irritability and increased aggressiveness to psy-chotic symptoms and full affective syndromes. Common reasons why these drugs are abused include to improve athletic performance and personal appearance (by increasing muscle mass). When the clinician suspects anabolic steroid abuse, urine screens for these drugs should be obtained, because not all patients will admit to steroid use. The abuse of these drugs can also be associated with liver abnormalities (e.g., liver enzyme elevations, increased bilirubin levels) and increases in low-density lipoproteins (LDLs).

Chronic high-dose *aspirin* (*salicylate*) use can cause tinnitus and even a possible organic hallucinosis. Patients on prescribed high-dose aspirin can have serum salicylate levels in the toxic range (greater than 20 mg/dl [1.45 mmol/liter]). Both aspirin and acetaminophen are commonly used in suicide overdose attempts, and sufficient doses of both can be quite lethal and require immediate medical attention.

■ REFERENCES

1. Frings CS, White RM, Battaglia DJ: Status of drugs-of-abuse testing in urine: an AACC study. Clin Chem 1987; 33:1683–1686
2. Panner MJ, Christakis NA: The limits of science in on-the-job screening. Hastings Cent Rep 1986; 16:6:7–12
3. Sramek JJ, Baumgartner WA, Tallos JA, et al: Hair analysis for detection of phencyclidine in newly admitted psychiatric patients. Am J Psychiatry 142:950–953, 1985
4. Ellenhorn MJ, Barceloux DG: Medical Toxicology: Diagnosis and Treatment of Human Poisoning. New York, Elsevier, 1988
5. Landrigan PJ, Baker D, Needleman HL: Lead poisoning in automobile radiator mechanics (letter). N Engl J Med 1988; 318:320
6. Goldman RH, Baker EL: Lead poisoning in automobile radiator mechanics (letter). N Engl J Med 1988; 318:320
7. Westermeyer J: The psychiatrist and solvent-inhalant abuse: recognition, assessment and treatment. Am J Psychiatry 1987; 144:903–907
8. Dager SR, Holland JP, Cowley DS, et al: Panic disorder precipitated by exposure to organic solvents in the work place. Am J Psychiatry 1987; 144:1056–1058

ADDITIONAL DIAGNOSTIC TESTS COMMONLY USED IN PSYCHIATRY 7

■ CHEST X RAY

The chest X ray is useful to the psychiatrist as part of the evaluation of the patient with potential cardiopulmonary disease (e.g., pneumonia, congestive heart failure). Such diseases can adversely affect mental functioning.

■ SKULL X RAY

The skull X ray can be used to help detect skull fractures, brain tumors (e.g., pituitary tumors), and other disease processes affecting the skull. In dementia workups, this test has largely been replaced by computed tomography (CT) of the head because CT can potentially detect pathology of the bony structures and brain parenchyma.

■ ELECTROCARDIOGRAM

The electrocardiogram (ECG or EKG) measures the electrical activity of the heart. Abnormalities of cardiac electrical activity signal cardiac pathology. The ECG is important to the psychiatrist 1) as part of the evaluation of possible cardiac dysfunction leading to problems with brain perfusion and 2) for monitoring possible adverse cardiac effects of commonly used psychotropic medications (e.g., tricyclic antidepressants). The ECG is also used in the evaluation of chest pain, coronary artery disease, cardiac arrhythmias, and electrolyte disturbances (e.g., low potassium). Very low serum potassium levels resulting in abnormal ECGs can be seen in the context of some eating disorders. The ECG can also be useful for detecting some substance-induced heart disease (e.g., secondary to cocaine).

A more thorough discussion of some of the ECG effects of psychotropic medications can be found in Chapter 8. The ECG is often an important component of the pretreatment and follow-up evaluation of a patient on psychotropic medications. Potentially serious cardiac complications of psychotropic therapy can be detected by ECG.

■ HOLTER MONITORING

A Holter monitor allows the patient's cardiac rhythm to be measured for hours (typically a full day) and while ambulatory during regular activity. Such monitoring is often employed in the workup of syncope, dizziness, and palpitations in the attempt to detect cardiac pathology (e.g., arrythmia, ST segment shifts) not seen in a routine resting ECG. The evaluation of panic disorder patients with cardiac symptoms can be assisted by Holter monitoring. Holter monitoring is sometimes referred to as ambulatory ECG.

■ ECHOCARDIOGRAPHY

Echocardiography (cardiac ultrasound) is commonly used in the evaluation of mitral-valve prolapse (MVP) or Barlow's syndrome. An association between MVP, anxiety, and panic disorders has been studied but never conclusively proven. For clinical management of anxious patients with possible MVP, Dager et al. (1) suggested that cardiac auscultation by an experienced and skilled clinician is perhaps more helpful than echocardiography. This usually involves consultation with an internist or cardiologist, who might or might not recommend further echocardiographic evaluation.

Other cardiac conditions that can be evaluated using echocardiography include cardiomyopathies, cardiac aneurysm, valvular disease in general, intracardiac masses, and endocarditis. Any of these disorders could ultimately compromise brain perfusion and lead to mental status abnormalities.

■ CAROTID ULTRASOUND

This test is sometimes included in a dementia workup, especially when multi-infarct dementia (MID) is suspected. The National Institute of Mental Health (NIMH) Consensus Conference on Dementia stated, however, that carotid ultrasound is of no value except in the search for possible causes of infarcts. Carotid ultrasound is used in the workup of transient ischemic attacks (TIAs) or stroke in evolution.

■ COMPUTED TOMOGRAPHY

Computed tomography (CT) scans are being increasingly ordered by psychiatrists to help rule out possible structural brain abnormalities that might be contributing to a patient's psychiatric presentation. Such brain abnormalities can include tumors, subdural hematomas, strokes, or brain abscesses. Table 7-1 lists some evolving indications for ordering a CT scan in psychiatric practice. Some clinicians might also utilize a CT in certain difficult treatment-resistant psychiatric patients to provide reassurance to patients and their families (as well as to the clinicians themselves) that no other brain pathology exists.

CT scanning of the head offers the clinician cross-sectional X-ray images of the brain from multiple brain levels (e.g., both cortical and subcortical brain regions). The CT can detect and

TABLE 7-1. Proposed Indications for Computed Tomography of the Head in Psychiatric Practice

Larson et al. (2)	Focal neurologic findings
Rosenberg et al. (3)	Abnormal electroencephalogram
Weinberger (4)	Unknown cases of • Confusion, dementia, delirium • First episode of psychosis • Movement disorder • Anorexia nervosa • Prolonged catatonia • First affective episode after age 50 • Personality change after age 50
Emsley et al. (5)	• Alcohol abuse • History of head trauma • History of seizures
Beresford et al. (6)	• Impaired cognition on mental status examination

image variations in tissue density and can provide a detailed structural view of brain tissue and skull. In addition to imaging the brain, the CT can be used to visualize the entire length of the spinal cord, as well as other body areas (e.g., abdomen, chest, neck).

A CT of the head typically exposes the patient to the same amount of radiation as a skull X-ray series. CT scans of the brain can be performed with or without contrast material. The intravenous injection of contrast media can be used to "enhance" the visualization of certain brain lesions (e.g., recent stroke, tumors, infections, and abscesses; processes that can interfere with the integrity of the blood-brain barrier), hence the term *contrast*—or *enhanced*—CT study. The decision as to whether contrast should be used is typically made by the radiologist. Adverse reactions to the contrast material can range from minor (e.g., a metallic taste sensation) to severe (e.g., an anaphylactic reaction with sudden cardiovascular collapse). Patients with histories of allergic reactions (e.g., to seafood, or asthma) have a greater chance of having an allergic reaction to the contrast material. The more expensive nonionic contrast media are associated with fewer allergic reactions. With some patients, radiologists might prophylactically treat them with steroids to decrease the likelihood of allergic reactions to the contrast dye. Note that radiologists sometimes use double-dose delayed CT (DDD-CT). In DDD-CT, approximately twice the ordinary dose of intravenous contrast material is used, and the actual x-raying of the brain is delayed compared with a conventional contrast CT. DDD-CT allows for better identification of certain brain lesions and can help to clarify ambiguous findings from a conventional single-dose CT contrast study.

Of course, the psychiatrist should rely on the expertise of the radiologist to direct a CT study properly.

STRUCTURAL ABNORMALITIES IN PSYCHIATRIC PATIENTS AS DETECTED BY CT

Research psychiatrists have used CT in an attempt to identify brain abnormalities in patients with idiopathic (functional) psychiatric disorder. Much of this work has focused on patients with schizophrenia. Findings in this area have included

1. A higher frequency of reversed cerebral asymmetry in patients with schizophrenia as compared with patients without schizophrenia (7),
2. Cerebellar atrophy and third ventricle enlargement in schizophrenic patients (8),
3. High ventricle-to-brain ratios (VBRs) in chronic schizophrenic and bipolar patients (9),
4. A negative correlation between ventricular enlargement and response to neuroleptic treatment in schizophrenic patients (10), and
5. More prefrontal markings (related to cortical atrophic changes) in schizophrenic patients than in normal controls (11).

However, the potential clinical meaning of these structural findings remains to be clarified.

THE CROW HYPOTHESIS

Crow proposed two different schizophrenic syndromes, Type I and Type II (12,13). Type I schizophrenia is associated with normal brain ventricular size on CT or magnetic resonance imaging (MRI), as well as "positive" symptoms of schizophrenia (e.g., delusions, hallucinations), a good response to neuroleptics, and a better prognosis. Type II schizophrenia is associated with enlarged ventricles, "negative" symptoms (e.g., blunted affect, poverty of speech), a poor response to neuroleptics, and a more chronic course (12, 13). However, potential overlap between the two syndromes has been noted: Type I schizophrenia reportedly can progress to Type II, and episodes of Type I can occur in a patient with a primarily Type II schizophrenic disorder (13).

However, several studies have not supported this hypothesis. Nevertheless, some psychiatrists have advocated using CT findings in selected treatment-resistant patients. Some have argued that high-dose neuroleptic treatment strategies might be pursued less vigorously in patients with predominantly negative symptoms demonstrating enlarged ventricles on CT, presumably on the basis that these Type II schizophrenic patients have a poorer response to neuroleptics, and it would not make sense to expose these patients to the potential dangers of this class of medications (e.g., tardive dyskinesia) in the face of expecting little benefit. However, this is an area of active research requiring further clarification before clear clinical strategies can be adopted. The main utility of CT in psychiatric patients at this time is to rule out other neurologic processes and not to make or refine our functional diagnoses. The research CT findings should help us to understand better the pathogenesis of schizophrenia and help us to generate hypotheses to be tested in the future.

■ MAGNETIC RESONANCE IMAGING

Like CT, magnetic resonance imaging (MRI) is used by psychiatrists in the evaluation of patients with suspected structural brain abnormality. Proposed indications for ordering MRI in psychiatric patients are similar to those proposed for CT (see Table 7-1) (14). Some lesions not well visualized by CT might be better detected and characterized by MRI. However, there are certain clinical situations where MRI is either contraindicated or nonoptimal compared with CT, and some investigators do not believe that MRI is "generally superior" to the less expensive and more widely available CT (15). MRI has also been referred to as nuclear magnetic resonance (NMR).

There are many different imaging modes available. Some best visualize anatomy, structure, and morphology; others emphasize particular characteristics of certain pathologic lesions. For instance, scanning modes providing what are referred to as "T_1 weighted images" are useful for visualizing brain anatomy and morphology. Edema on a T_1 weighted image looks dark (hypodense). Scanning modes providing "T_2 weighted images" visualize white matter pathology very well. Edema on a T_2 weighted image looks white (hyperdense). The uses of some scanning modes, pulse sequences, and MRI contrast agents are still under investigation.

■ COMPARISON OF CT AND MRI

CT is currently more available to most practicing clinicians than MRI. The cost of a single CT scan for an individual patient is still lower than for an MRI scan. Table 7-2 lists certain situa-

TABLE 7-2. **Magnetic Resonance Imaging (MRI) Instead of Computed Tomography (CT)**

Anatomic regions suspected:
- Temporal lobes
- Cerebellum
- Subcortical structures
- Brain stem
- Spinal cord

Particular disease suspected:
- White matter of demyelinating disorders
- Seizure focus
- Dementia
- Infarction
- Neoplasm (other than meningeal)
- Vascular malformation (including angiographically occult)
- Huntington's disease (and other degenerative disease)

Children (posterior fossa, temporal lobe, midline)

CT contraindicated to avoid:
- Radiation
- Iodine-based contrast material
- Intravenous procedure

Note. Reproduced with permission from Garber HJ, Weinberg JB, Buonanno FS, et al: Use of magnetic resonance imaging in psychiatry. Am J Psychiatry 1988; 145:164–171. Copyright 1988 American Psychiatric Association.

tions where an MRI might be ordered instead of a CT scan (e.g., for patients in whom a contrast CT study is needed but who are allergic to the iodine-based contrast material). Table 7-3 outlines situations where a CT scan might be superior to an MRI (e.g., patients in whom an MRI is contraindicated due to pregnancy). Table 7-4 lists potential patient scenarios where an MRI might be ordered after a CT has already been performed.

The reader should be aware that this is an evolving area. More work will be needed to decide when MRI or CT is most appropriate. Indeed, the use of new contrast agents for MRI might introduce some new indications for MRI. Consultation with a neurologist or neuroradiologist would help the psychiatrist trying to choose between MRI and CT for a particular patient and serves to maximize the usefulness of these studies in a psychiatric patient.

TABLE 7-3. **Computed Tomography (CT) Instead of Magnetic Resonance Imaging (MRI)**

No localizing abnormalities present

No specific disease suspected that would be better evaluated with MRI

Suspected pathology well studied in CT
- Meningeal tumor (primary or metastatic)
- Pituitary lesions
- Calcified lesions
- Acute subarachnoid or parenchymal hemorrhage
- Acute parenchymal infarction

MRI contraindicated due to
- Pacemaker
- Aneurysm clip
- Ferromagnetic foreign body
- Pregnancy

Note. Reproduced with permission from Garber HJ, Weinberg JB, Buonanno FS, et al: Use of magnetic resonance imaging in psychiatry. Am J Psychiatry 1988; 145:164–171. Copyright 1988 American Psychiatric Association.

TABLE 7-4. **Magnetic Resonance Imaging (MRI) after Computed Tomography (CT)**

CT abnormal but not diagnostic

Equivocal or normal CT but high index of suspicion for disease likely to be seen better with MRI

Normal CT but atypical symptoms or course

Normal CT but strong clinical or emotional need for reassurance with MRI

Note. Reproduced with permission from Garber HJ, Weinberg JB, Buonanno FS, et al: Use of magnetic resonance imaging in psychiatry. Am J Psychiatry 1988; 145:164–171. Copyright 1988 American Psychiatric Association.

■ THE ELECTROENCEPHALOGRAM

The electroencephalogram (EEG) is an important tool for the clinical psychiatrist in the differentiation of psychiatric and organic mental disorders. Organic conditions that can be evaluated with the help of the EEG include epilepsy, central nervous system (CNS) tumor, trauma, stroke, degenerative conditions, and disordered metabolic states causing delirium. The EEG measures brain electrical activity originating from neurons located primarily in the uppermost cortical cell layers of the brain. This electrical activity is measured from electrodes placed on the scalp in standardized positions (conforming to the international 10-20 system of scalp electrode placement). The electrical activity is recorded as waves of varying frequencies and amplitudes. EEG frequencies have been divided into the following bands: beta activity ($\geq$13 Hz), alpha rhythm (8 to 12 Hz), theta activity (4 to 7 Hz), and delta activity ($<$4 Hz).

ABNORMAL EEG FINDINGS

Abnormal EEG findings can be divided into a number of different categories (16):

1. *Dysrhythmia.* This can include abnormal bursts of spikes, sharp waves, or slow activity. Spike or sharp waves are pointed peaks on an EEG recording that are transient and stand out from the rest of the EEG record. A spike is typically defined as having a duration of less than 80 msec; sharp waves are generally considered as having durations greater than 80 msec. Note that the absence of dysrhythmia on an EEG recording does not rule out the possible presence of seizure activity in a patient. Indeed, the EEG does not have absolute sensitivity for detecting underlying seizure disorders. For instance, the paroxysmal electrical activity responsible for a certain clinical presentation may not always occur during the time of the EEG recording. When sampling error is suspected and the suspicion of some seizure disorder is high, possible interventions that can be employed to detect clinically significant dysrhythmia more accurately can include 1) repeat EEGs, 2) sleep–deprived EEGs, or 3) 24-hour ambulatory EEG recordings, which can be accompanied by a video recording in an attempt to further document possible seizure activity.
2. *EEG slow wave activity.* Clinically significant slowing includes the presence of theta or delta activity recorded while the patient is awake. This can be seen in many cases of delirium and in some cases of dementia. In fact, a slow EEG (i.e.,

an awake EEG with prominent theta or delta activity) is often cited as being useful in differentiating the delirious patient from a patient with an idiopathic (i.e., functional) psychiatric illness. However, delirium due to withdrawal from alcohol or sedative-hypnotic drugs is typically associated with excessive background fast activity. Psychoactive medications potentially associated with EEG slowing include lithium, phenothiazines, benzodiazepines, tricyclics, anticonvulsants, and narcotics.

3. *EEG amplitude suppression.* Conditions in which this can be seen include brain death and subdural hematoma. Subdural hematomas can present with mental status changes and complicate alcohol withdrawal and degenerative brain disease.

4. *EEG asymmetries.* For example, when comparing EEG voltages and frequencies from homologous regions of the left and right sides of the scalp, asymmetries can be of clinical significance (i.e., suggest focal brain disease). EEG asymmetries have been reported in certain functional psychiatric disorders (e.g., depression, mania, schizophrenia); however, the clinical significance of such findings is unclear at this time.

UNMASKING LATENT ABNORMAL EEG ACTIVITY

Abnormal EEG activity is not always detected by simply attaching electrodes to a patient's scalp and recording the EEG. Certain procedures are often utilized in an attempt to unmask latent abnormal EEG activity. These can include photic stimulation and hyperventilation as well as sleep deprivation, use of nasopharyngeal (NP) leads, evoked potentials, and computerized EEG recordings.

Photic stimulation is a common form of provocative stimulation where the patient is exposed to a flashing strobe light during the EEG recording. Abnormal "photoconvulsive" responses are manifested by paroxysmal EEG activity that is not synchronized with the flashing of the strobe light.

Hyperventilation is another form of provocative EEG testing. The patient is typically asked to hyperventilate for about three minutes. Abnormal EEG responses to such a procedure can include the appearance of spike or sharp waves or the appearance of paroxysms of slow wave activity.

SLEEP-DEPRIVED EEG RECORDINGS

After sleep deprivation, certain abnormalities are more likely to become manifest during an EEG recording. The sleep deprivation makes it more likely that the patient will fall asleep during the procedure, and it is during the changes in the level of consciousness while falling asleep that certain EEG abnormalities (e.g., spike and sharp wave activity) are more likely to become manifest. The clinician should check with the EEG laboratory to find out the specific protocol employed for sleep deprivation so that the patient can be provided with proper instructions for staying up the night prior to the EEG. Many EEG laboratories prefer to do a non-sleep-deprived EEG prior to ordering a sleep-deprived EEG. Hall et al. (17) felt that the sleep-deprived EEG for psychiatric patients is more sensitive than a routine, non-sleep-deprived EEG.

NASOPHARYNGEAL LEADS

It has been suggested that the use of nasopharyngeal (NP) leads in psychiatric patients can increase the diagnostic yield of the EEG recording (18). Grebb et al. (19) suggested using both sleep deprivation and NP leads in the workup of a newly diagnosed psychotic patient. A study by Ramani et al. (20) questioned the value of NP leads, especially when the NP leads are uncomfortable enough to interfere with the patient trying to fall asleep after sleep deprivation. Sleep deprivation with subsequent sleep during the EEG recording is considered by some to be more valuable diagnostically than the utilization of NP leads (20). Currently, there is no complete consensus about the value of the EEG supplemented with NP leads in psychiatric patients. The reader should note, however, that there have been patients in whom abnormal EEG activity has been seen only with NP leads.

APPLICATION OF THE EEG IN PSYCHIATRY

The EEG is most commonly used by psychiatrists to help differentiate some organic brain disorders (e.g., seizure disorders, delirium, and dementia) from functional psychiatric conditions. Lam et al. (21) reported that the clinical situations most associated with abnormal EEGs in a population of psychiatric inpatients were a seizure disorder history or suspicion of a recent seizure, or when there was a strong suspicion of organic mental disease based on history or physical or mental status examination. They reported that no unexpected organic disease was detected by EEG in the psychiatric inpatients they studied, hence their recommendations against the automatic, routine use of the EEG for psychiatric patients. They recommended that the EEG be used as a supplemental test in patients whose history and other clinical findings are already suggestive of organic mental disease. Some authors have suggested that patients with a history of episodic behavioral or mental disturbance should have an EEG study.

Figure 7-1 outlines a possible strategy for ordering an EEG in a psychiatric patient. Again, a normal EEG does not exclude the possibility that the patient has a seizure disorder, or any other organic disease for that matter. As Lam et al. (21) pointed out, the sensitivity and specificity for the EEG are best in seizure disorder and delirium, and much lower for other brain diseases such as dementia, strokes, tumors, or subdural hematomas.

The EEG is not considered useful in identifying specific functional psychiatric disorders. Although an increased number of nonspecific EEG abnormalities have been noted in a variety of psychiatric disorders (e.g., schizophrenia), none of these are considered diagnostic or of clinical utility in diagnosing functional psychiatric disturbances at this time. Another area of growing interest is pharmacoelectroencephalography (PEEG), which involves the study of how various psychotropic medications and drugs affect the EEG.

■ EVOKED POTENTIALS

Evoked potential (EP) testing is an extension of conventional EEG recording. Like the EEG, EPs can assist the psychiatrist or neurologist in the differentiation between some "organic" and "functional" (i.e., idiopathic) complaints (e.g., in the differentiation between hysterical versus organic blindness using visual EP testing). Additionally, EP testing has established uses in clinical

History of: Physical exam shows:

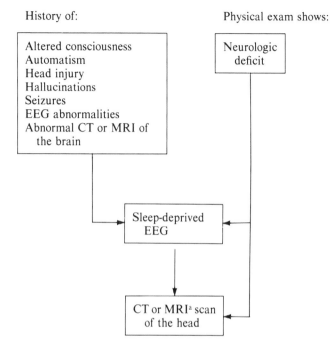

FIGURE 7–1. **Strategy for obtaining an EEG in a psychiatric patient to rule out temporal lobe epilepsy**

Adapted from Raj A, Sheehan DV: Medical evaluation of panic attacks. J Clin Psychiatry 1987; 48:309–313. With permission from publisher. Copyright 1987 Physicians Postgraduate Press. ªMRI may be superior to CT for detecting brain abnormalities related to seizure foci in patients with partial seizure syndromes.

neurology and neurosurgical practice, including uses in the evaluation of demyelinating disorders such as multiple sclerosis and in the intraoperative evaluation of nerve functioning during certain neurosurgical procedures. Although some types of EP peculiarities have been noted in certain psychiatric disorders, none are considered to be of clear clinical utility at this time. For example, the P-300 is an EP that occurs in most subjects about 300 msec after the presentation and perception of a novel stimulus (e.g., a tone or visual image). Delayed and smaller P-300 responses have been noted in patients with schizophrenia and borderline personality disorder (22).

THE EP TEST

In EP testing, brain EEG responses to specific sensory stimuli are measured. The evoking stimulus can be 1) auditory, as in auditory EP (AEP) or in brain stem AEP (BSAEP); 2) visual (VEP); or 3) somatosensory (SSEP), typically accomplished with brief electrical stimuli delivered to an extremity (e.g., to the tibial or median nerves).

In the process of EP testing, the subject is repeatedly exposed to these stimuli. For example, in the case of VEP, the stimuli might involve flashing lights or an alternating checkerboard pattern. The evoked EEG responses are measured in a manner similar to a conventional EEG recording (e.g., using the international 10-20 system of electrode placement). The multiple evoked brain electrical responses are then added together and averaged by a computer. By doing this, the computer is able to remove most of the background, non–stimulus-related activity, and the computer-generated result is a characteristic EP waveform. This EP waveform typically consists of positive and negative peaks spread out over a time axis measured in milliseconds. Early peaks are generally defined as those EP peaks occurring within the first 50 msec poststimulus; late peaks occur after 250 msec. An example of an early EP is the BSAEP; middle peaks include the N100-P200 complex. Late peaks include the P300, the contingent negative variation (CNV), the post-imperative negative variation (PINV), the movement-related potential (MRP), and the selective attention effect (Nd). The CNV and PINV can be measured for up to several seconds after certain stimuli; the MRP is thought to reflect preparation for movement and typically occurs between 500 and 1,000 msec after the subject is signaled to move. The Nd is associated with attention to a stimulus and can be seen from about 60 to 500 msec after the stimulus. The usefulness of any of these EPs in the diagnosis of psychiatric disorder, however, is still under investigation.

■ COMPUTERIZED TOPOGRAPHIC MAPPING OF EEG AND EP DATA

In the computerized topographic mapping of EEG and EP data, computers are used to amass and process large quantities of EEG and EP data and to present these data graphically in ways useful to the psychiatrist. Typically, the computers analyze the data in various ways and present the results in two-dimensional, color-coded maps of brain electrical activity. Several manufacturers currently offer computerized EEG and EP equipment; the capabilities and methods of data analysis vary between manufacturers. There are several problems associated with the computerized EEG and EP systems currently available: 1) standardization is lacking between products, 2) the normative data for the different systems are of varying quality, 3) maps obtained on different machines are not always comparable, and 4) different products use differing statistical approaches to generate their maps. The current American Electroencephalographic Society (AEEGS) recommendation regards computerized topographic mapping as primarily a research tool at this time; hence, clinical applications are limited and adjunctive. The AEEGS recommends that standard EEG and EP studies done according to AEEGS guidelines should accompany computerized EEG and EP reports.

■ POLYSOMNOGRAPHY

Psychiatrists are becoming increasingly involved in the evaluation of patients with various sleep disorders, including insomnia, parasomnias, narcolepsy, and sleep apnea. Polysomnography is often an important part of such an evaluation. As the "poly" in polysomnography implies, multiple physiologic measures are typically made during a polysomnogram, including 1) a recording of EEG activity during sleep or attempts at sleep (the sleep EEG); 2) electro-oculograms (EOGs), which are used to assist in the differentiation of rapid eye movement (REM) sleep from nonrapid eye movement (NREM) sleep; 3) electromyograms (EMG), to assist in the evaluation of nocturnal myoclonus and the evaluation of REM sleep, which is typically associated with a reduction in muscle tone; and 4) ECG (useful in the evaluation of the cardiovascular effects of sleep apnea). Apnea can be associated with cardiac arrhythmias, bradycardia, or tachycardia.

Other polysomnographic measures include blood oxygen saturation (e.g., with ear oximeter), respiratory effort (e.g., by the use of strain gauges located at the abdomen and chest), air flow (e.g., by measuring air movement at the nose and mouth), and blood pressure (BP) recordings (BP becomes more variable during REM sleep and can become quite elevated during periods of sleep apnea). Other measures such as time asleep and body temperature are typically made. (REM sleep is associated with some loss of thermoregulation.)

POSSIBLE INDICATIONS FOR SLEEP EEG OR POLYSOMNOGRAPHY IN PSYCHIATRIC PATIENTS

There is incomplete consensus regarding the indications for a sleep EEG or polysomnography in psychiatric patients. Jacobs et al. (23) recommended that polysomnography be done in patients with chronic insomnia who have been "treatment resistant" (i.e., have failed to respond to routine treatment interventions, including attempts at improving "sleep hygiene" or removing factors that can interfere with sleep). Jacobs et al. (23) presented evidence suggesting that polysomnography can be of great assistance in clarifying the etiology of a patient's complaint of chronic insomnia.

Some investigators have used the sleep EEG as a marker of endogenous depression. Proposed sleep EEG markers include a shortened REM latency (usually less than 65 minutes) and increased REM density. Other possible sleep EEG markers of depression include sleep continuity disturbances and diminished slow wave sleep activity (i.e., decreased stages 3 and 4 sleep), as well as altered distribution of REM sleep activity. Recent research (24) reported that patients with mania tend to demonstrate EEG sleep findings similar to those found in patients with depression (i.e., shortened REM latency, increased REM activity, and increased REM density).

Patients with neuromedical disorders (e.g., endocrinopathies) have been reported as demonstrating greatly decreased REM activity and REM density. Patients who demonstrate such findings during a workup of a sleep disorder might be best served by a thorough search for medical disorders contributing to the patient's insomnia or psychiatric condition (23). Reynolds et al. (25) suggested that the sleep EEG can help in the differential diagnosis between depression and dementia. They reported four measures that helped to discriminate between depression and dementia: 1) shorter REM latency in the patients with depression, 2) higher percentage of REM sleep in depressed patients, 3) higher percentage of non-REM sleep in the patients with dementia, and 4) more marked early morning awakening in the depressed patients.

Nocturnal polysomnography is also used in the evaluation of sleep apnea, somnambulism (sleepwalking disorder), parvor nocturnus (sleep-terror disorder), enuresis, nightmares (dream anxiety disorder), and bruxism. In the case of sleep apnea, polysomnography is important in the differentiation between obstructive versus central sleep apnea. In the case of obstructive apnea, continuous positive airway pressure (CPAP), which eliminates the airway occlusion, can be utilized during a polysomnographic recording to see if improvement in blood oxygen saturation can be obtained.

The multiple sleep latency test (MSLT) is a special daytime sleep evaluation for narcolepsy. Because a single normal sleep EEG does not rule out narcolepsy, multiple recordings might need to be made. Note that narcolepsy is only one type of hypersomnia. The differential diagnosis of hypersomnia can be extensive and can include psychiatric disorders, sleep apnea, nocturnal myoclonus, or "restless legs" syndrome.

■ NOCTURNAL PENILE TUMESCENCE TESTS

Nocturnal penile tumescence (NPT) tests involve the evaluation of erectile function during sleep. Penile erections are associated with REM sleep and are typically unrelated to any erotic dream content. NPT studies are helpful, although not completely reliable, in the differentiation between organic versus functional causes of impotence (26). For example, abnormal NPT studies suggestive of an organic etiology for impotence have been reported in depression (27). NPT tests can be completed as part of a polysomnographic evaluation.

NPT tests generally involve the quantification of such parameters as penile circumference changes (e.g., by strain gauges placed at the base and tip of the penis), penile rigidity (which measures the force that causes the erect penis to buckle), and the frequency of penile tumescence during sleep. A typical NPT test includes two to three nights of recording. Portable NPT recording systems that can be used either in the sleep laboratory or in the patient's home are available.

■ REFERENCES

1. Dager SR, Comess KA, Dunner DL: Mitral valve prolapse and anxiety disorders. Hosp Community Psychiatry 1988; 39:517–527
2. Larson EB, Reifler BV, Sumi SM, et al: Diagnostic tests in the evaluation of dementia: a prospective study of 200 elderly outpatients. Arch Intern Med 1986; 146:1917–1922
3. Rosenberg CE, Anderson DC, Mahowald MW, et al: Computed tomography and EEG in patients without focal neurologic findings. Arch Neurol 1982; 39:291–292
4. Weinberger DR: Brain disease and psychiatric illness: when should a psychiatrist order a CT scan? Am J Psychiatry 1984; 141:1521–1527
5. Emsley RA, Gledhill RF, Bell PS, et al: Indications for CAT scans of psychiatric patients (letter). Am J Psychiatry 1986; 143:1199
6. Beresford TP, Blow FC, Nicholos LO, et al: Focal signs and brain CT scans in psychiatric patients. N Engl J Med 1986; 313:388
7. Luchins DJ, Weinberger DR, Wyatt RJ: Schizophrenia: evidence of a subgroup with reversed cerebral asymmetry. Arch Gen Psychiatry 1979; 36:1309–1311
8. Nasrallah HA, Jacoby CO, Chapman J, et al: Third ventricle enlargement on CT scan in schizophrenia: association with cerebellar atrophy. Biol Psychiatry 1985; 20:443–450
9. Pearlson GD, Garbacz DJ, Breakey WR, et al: Lateral ventricular enlargement associated with persistent unemployment and negative symptoms in both schizophrenia and bipolar disorder. Psychiatry Res 1984; 12:1–9
10. Weinberger DR, Bigelow LB, Kleinman JF, et al: Cerebral ventricular enlargement in chronic schizophrenia: an association with poor response to treatment. Arch Gen Psychiatry 1980; 37:22–23
11. Shelton RC, Karson CN, Doran AR, et al: Cerebral structure pathology in schizophrenia: evidence for a selective prefrontal cortical defect. Am J Psychiatry 1988; 145:154–163
12. Crow TJ: Positive and negative schizophrenia symptoms and the role of dopamine. Br J Psychiatry 1981; 139:251–264

13. Bird J, Harrison G: Examination Notes in Psychiatry, 2nd ed. Bristol, England, IOP Publishing Limited, Techno House, 1987

14. Garber HJ, Weinberg JB, Buonanno FS, et al: Use of magnetic resonance imaging in psychiatry. Am J Psychiatry 1988; 145:164–171

15. Kent DL, Larson EB: Magnetic resonance imaging of the brain and spine. Ann Intern Med 1988; 108:402–424

16. Nunez PL: Electric Fields of the Brain: The Neurophysics of EEG. New York, Oxford University Press, 1981

17. Hall RCW, Gardner ER, Stickney SK, et al: Physical illness manifesting as psychiatric disease. Arch Gen Psychiatry 1980; 376:989–995

18. Sternberg DE: Testing for physical illness in psychiatric patients. J Clin Psychiatry 1986; 47(suppl):3–9

19. Grebb JA, Weinberger DR, Morihisa JM: Electroencephalogram and evoked potential studies of schizophrenia, in Handbook of Schizophrenia, vol 1: The Neurology of Schizophrenia. New York, Elsevier, 1986

20. Ramani V, Loewenson RB, Torrey F: The limited usefulness of nasopharyngeal EEG recording in psychiatric patients. Am J Psychiatry 1985; 142:1099–1100

21. Lam RW, Hurwitz TA, Wada JA: The clinical use of EEG in a general psychiatric setting. Hosp Community Psychiatry 1988; 39:533–536

22. Kutcher SP, Blackwood SH, St Clair D, et al: Auditory P-300 in borderline personality disorder and schizophrenia. Arch Gen Psychiatry 1987; 44:645–650

23. Jacobs EA, Reynolds CF, Kupfer DJ, et al: The role of polysomnography in the differential diagnosis of chronic insomnia. Ann J Psychiatry 1988; 145:346–349

24. Hudson JI, Lipinski JR, Frankenburg FR: Electroencephalographic sleep in mania. Arch Gen Psychiatry 1988; 45:267–273

25. Reynolds CF, Kupfer DJ, Houck PR, et al: Reliable discrimination of elderly depressed and demented patients by electroencephalographic sleep data. Arch Gen Psychiatry 1988; 45:258–264

26. Thase ME, Reynolds CF, Glanz LM, et al: Nocturnal penile tumescence in depressed men. Am J Psychiatry 1987; 144:80–92

27. Williams W: Psychogenic erectile impotence: a useful or a misleading concept? Aust NZ J Psychiatry 1985; 19:77–82

8 LABORATORY AND DIAGNOSTIC TESTS FOR SOMATIC THERAPIES IN PSYCHIATRY

One of the major uses of the clinical laboratory for the psychiatrist includes helping guard the patient being treated with organic therapies against some of the potential toxicities of these therapies. These toxicities can range from subclinical to potentially fatal. The tests ordered in the context of organic psychiatric treatments can be divided into *pretreatment* and *follow-up* laboratory and diagnostic tests. Pretreatment evaluations provide a baseline for future comparison and help to detect those patients who might be most susceptible to certain adverse reactions to the organic treatments proposed. Follow-up evaluations help to identify those patients experiencing untoward medical side effects from the organic treatments being used. Additionally, for some psychotropic medications, *therapeutic blood levels* have been proposed, and the follow-up evaluations might include determinations of these medication blood levels.

■ TRICYCLIC ANTIDEPRESSANTS

MEDICAL PRETREATMENT AND FOLLOW-UP LABORATORY EVALUATIONS

No universally accepted medical pretreatment and follow-up laboratory evaluation protocols have been developed for the tricyclic antidepressants (TCAs). Gelenberg (1) recommended a medical laboratory evaluation strategy based on the individual patient's past medical history, physical examination, previous history of adverse drug reactions, and knowledge of the potential side effects of the TCAs. For instance, liver function tests might be ordered in a patient with a history of liver disease who is about to be started on a TCA. In such a patient, liver function tests might need to be followed periodically throughout the patient's treatment. The patient who becomes delirious while on a TCA would need a careful workup for an organic mental disorder (potentially TCA induced), which might include an electroencephalogram (EEG), electrocardiogram (ECG), and TCA blood level. (Note that TCAs and the tetracyclic antidepressant maprotiline reportedly lower seizure thresholds.)

ECG CHANGES ASSOCIATED WITH TCAs

In a patient about to be started on a TCA, an ECG is typically ordered if the patient has a history of cardiac pathology because TCAs are sometimes associated with ECG changes. TCAs can increase heart rate; their anticholinergic effect is primarily responsible for this. Other changes can include prolongation of the PR, QT, or QRS intervals, as well as ST- and T-wave changes. Arrhythmias have been seen in patients taking various TCAs; however, the action of the TCAs on the heart is thought to resemble Type I antiarrythmics (e.g., quinidine, procainamide). The TCAs can exacerbate or cause atrioventricular (AV) or bundle branch block. It is believed that when the QT interval corrected for rate (QTc) exceeds about 0.440 seconds in a patient on a TCA, there is an increased risk of sudden cardiac death due to malignant arrhythmias such as ventricular tachycardia or ventricular fibrillation (2). Patients who seem at particularly high risk of developing potentially lethal arrhythmias are those patients with preexisting prolonged QT intervals, those with excessive QT prolongation acquired during TCA treatment (3), and those with preexisting conduction abnormalities such as second-degree heart block and bifascicular block. The risk to patients with more stable forms of heart block (e.g., left or right bundle branch block) is not clear, but a certain amount of caution in these patients seems wise. Patients on both a Type I antiarrhythmic and a TCA should be monitored closely. Although moderate prolongations of PR, QRS, and QTc intervals are not absolute contraindications to TCA treatment, patients with such prolongations need close monitoring. Additionally, the nontricyclic antidepressant trazodone has anecdotally been associated with the generation of certain arrhythmias (ventricular ectopy); maprotiline with ventricularic tachycardia; and the newer TCA amoxapine with atrial flutter and fibrillation.

In the absence of a history of cardiac pathology, Gelenberg (1) suggested obtaining an ECG in a man over age 30 or a woman over age 40 who is about to start on a TCA and has not had an ECG in the past year. The initial ECG would provide a baseline to which future ECGs could be compared. In the pretreatment ECG, careful attention should be paid to evidence of conduction delay (i.e., QTc greater than .440 seconds, QRS greater than 0.11 seconds) and AV or bundle branch block. In the context of a TCA overdose, certain emergency physicians have reported that a widened QRS (i.e., greater than 0.10 seconds) can be more reliable for predicting the degree of potential TCA-induced cardiac toxicity and morbidity than an antidepressant blood level (4). Also in the context of TCA overdose, many different rhythm disturbances are possible.

THERAPEUTIC ANTIDEPRESSANT BLOOD LEVELS

In a group of patients on a fixed dose of antidepressant medication, a surprisingly wide range of plasma levels can be found. Hence, it is difficult to predict what antidepressant dose will be sufficient for an individual patient. Some patients on seemingly low or very conservative doses of a TCA can have remarkably high plasma levels of the medication, making them more susceptible to potential adverse effects. Conversely, some patients on high doses of a TCA can have low blood levels, making them less likely to have a therapeutic response to the TCA.

The American Psychiatric Association (APA) Task Force on the Use of Laboratory Tests in Psychiatry (5) stated that "plasma level measurements of imipramine, desmethylimipramine (desipramine), and nortriptyline are unequivocally useful in certain situations." Potential situations include when

1. Patients show questionable compliance;
2. Patients have a poor response to a "typical" antidepressant dose;
3. There is a need to obtain a potentially therapeutic dose of a TCA as rapidly as possible because of severe illness (e.g., with a severely suicidal patient);
4. Patients need the lowest potentially effective dose of the TCA

because of particular sensitivity to side effects (e.g., because of medical illness or age); and

5. Patients experience side effects at a very low dose.

The clinician might also want to check a TCA blood level in a patient who initially responded to a TCA but then experienced a breakthrough depression. Furthermore, Siris (6) suggested that patients taking a TCA concomitantly with a neuroleptic should have a TCA plasma concentration checked because TCAs and neuroleptics can reportedly interfere with each others' metabolism. Unexpectedly high TCA levels have been reported in some patients taking a concomitant neuroleptic. Additionally, TCA blood levels can reportedly change when the brand of TCA is switched (e.g., from brand name to generic). This is presumably related to differences in the bioavailability of the different preparations.

RECOMMENDED THERAPEUTIC BLOOD LEVELS

Therapeutic blood levels described by the APA Task Force (5) are listed in Table 8-1. Therapeutic blood levels for antidepressants other than those listed, including other TCAs (e.g., amitriptyline or doxepin) and nontricyclic antidepressants (e.g., maprotiline or trazodone), have been reported, but their utility is still under investigation. Certain hospital and commercial laboratories sometimes describe slightly different therapeutic levels than outlined in Table 8-1, and some will describe some preliminarily established "therapeutic" plasma levels for antidepressants besides the three TCAs listed in Table 8-1. Indeed, there is some disagreement about which plasma TCA levels are associated with optimal therapeutic response for all the antidepressants, including the TCAs. Good clinical judgment should be the final arbiter for antidepressant dose changes.

Samples for TCA blood levels are typically drawn about 12 hours after the last dose of the TCA (e.g., in the morning after the last nighttime dose). Additionally, steady-state blood levels for the TCAs are generally achieved after five half-lives of the TCA have passed (which is usually around 10 days after initiating the medication or changing the medication dose). Hence, TCA levels are typically drawn about 10 days after being on the same dose of

TABLE 8-1. **Tricyclic Antidepressant (TCA) Therapeutic Levels Suggested by APA Task Force on the Use of Laboratory Tests in Psychiatry**

TCA	Blood Levels
Imipramine	Total of imipramine + desmethylimipramine (desipramine) > 200 ng/ml
Nortriptyline	50–150 ng/ml ("therapeutic window")
Desipramine	> 125 ng/ml

Note. American Psychiatric Association Task Force on the Use of Laboratory Tests in Psychiatry: Tricyclic antidepressants—blood level measurements and clinical outcome: an APA Task Force Report. Am J Psychiatry 1985; 142:155–162. Copyright 1985 American Psychiatric Association.

the medication, as the levels described as therapeutic in the literature are steady–state blood levels.

For use of the TCAs or other antidepressants to treat psychiatric disorders other than depression (e.g., panic attacks, certain chronic pain conditions, nightmares related to posttraumatic stress disorder), therapeutic blood levels have not yet been defined. An interesting study by Lydiard (7) suggested that in agoraphobia with panic attacks, desipramine plasma levels above approximately 125 ng/ml seem to provide the greatest antipanic efficacy. Therefore, at least for desipramine, the therapeutic blood level that has been established for major depression seems to be similar to the therapeutic blood level that has been preliminarily suggested as most effective in panic disorder.

■ LITHIUM

The initial laboratory workup helps provide useful baseline data for the patient about to begin treatment with lithium. Lithium can have several potentially significant adverse effects, including those on the kidney, thyroid gland, heart, and developing fetus. Table 8-2 outlines some important pretreatment lithium laboratory determinations. Note that lithium is commonly associated with a benign elevation of the white blood cell (WBC) count (the leukocytosis is typically in the range of 10,000 to 15,000 cells/mm³); this WBC elevation can sometimes be confused with or mask an underlying infectious process.

TABLE 8-2. **Some Important Pretreatment Lithium Laboratory Determinations**

- Complete blood count
- Serum electrolytes
- Blood urea nitrogen [a]
- Serum creatinine [a]
- Thyroid function tests (e.g., TSH, T_3RU, T_4) [a]
- Antithyroid antibodies [b]
- Urinalysis
- Electrocardiogram [a]
- Pregnancy test in potentially childbearing women
- 24-hour urine for creatinine clearance and protein [a,c]

Note. TSH = thyroid-stimulating hormone; T_3RU = triiodothyronine resin uptake; T_4 = thyroxine.

[a] In addition to serum lithium levels, these tests are often employed in periodic follow-up evaluations of patients taking lithium. However, other tests should be ordered if clinically indicated in a particular lithium-treated patient.

[b] Possibly predictive of lithium-induced hypothyroidism. Utility in this regard, however, has yet to be clearly determined.

[c] Especially in patients with a history of kidney abnormalities or dysfunction, or patients who develop such abnormalities or dysfunction while on lithium.

Thyroid function tests commonly obtained include thyroid-stimulating hormone (TSH), triiodothyronine resin uptake (T_3RU), and thyroxine (T_4) tests. Thyroid changes that have been described with lithium therapy include a small drop in serum T_4 values after about six months of lithium treatment, usually returning to pretreatment levels within 12 months (8). After 12 months, T_4 levels have been reported to increase to above baseline. TSH levels have been reported to increase during the first year or so. Importantly, patients with past histories of thyroid illness have been reported to experience greater changes in both T_4 and TSH compared with patients without such histories. All in all, abnormal thyroid function tests may occur in 5 to 15 percent of patients treated with long-term lithium therapy. However, clinically significant thyroid disease secondary to lithium treatment is believed to be rare (8). Any patient on lithium with clinical signs or symptoms suggestive of thyroid disease (e.g., weight gain, fatigue, asthenia, cold intolerance, skin or voice changes) should have their thyroid functioning checked (see Figure 2-1). For patients taking lithium, regular monitoring of TSH levels every six to 12 months is probably sufficient laboratory follow-up. However, the frequency and extent of thyroid testing should also be directed by the patient's personal or family history of thyroid disease and by the presence of abnormal or borderline baseline thyroid function values. After lithium discontinuation, laboratory changes that have been reported include increases in mean thyroid indices (T_3, free T_4, and T_4); decreases in mean serum levels of calcium, magnesium, potassium, cholesterol, and triglycerides; and decreases in the WBC and red blood cell (RBC) counts (9).

The measurement of serum free T_4 (fT_4) in the thyroid evaluation of lithium-treated patients is being increasingly advocated; it is believed to be a more sensitive indicator of thyroid dysfunction than the currently more frequently used serum T_4 (10). The measurement of fT_4 has become technically easier and is becoming more commercially available. Additionally, lithium-associated hypothyroidism is thought to be linked to the presence of preexisting Hashimoto's thyroiditis; hence some clinicians utilize antithyroid antibodies as part of a prelithium workup. Finally, parathyroid dysfunction has also rarely been associated with lithium treatment. Some indications for obtaining parathormone levels in these patients are outlined in Figure 2-1.

Other tests that are recommended in the laboratory evaluation of the patient treated with lithium include a blood urea nitrogen (BUN), serum creatinine, urinalysis, and serum electrolytes (especially serum sodium). A more extensive panel of kidney function tests, including a 24-hour urine volume, creatinine clearance, and protein excretion, are typically obtained in patients with a history of kidney disease or if the expectation is that the patient will be on lithium long-term. Lithium treatment can slightly decrease glucose tolerance; hence a fasting blood sugar (FBS) is often obtained. Importantly, for potentially pregnant women, a pregnancy test should be ordered to rule out pregnancy.

ECG changes associated with lithium include T-wave flattening or inversion (generally reversible with the discontinuation of lithium) and, more rarely, evidence of sinus node dysfunction (e.g., sinus bradycardia, sinoatrial block, sinus arrest, and asystole). Other arrhythmias (e.g., supraventricular and ventricular tachyarrhythmias) have also been reported in patients taking lithium; whether these are related to lithium intake is unclear. An ECG should be obtained in a patient with a history or physical exam suggestive of cardiac disease. Brady and Hogan (11) recommended baseline ECGs in all lithium-treated patients with preexisting cardiac disease and those on other cardiotoxic medications.

LABORATORY AND DIAGNOSTIC TESTING DURING MAINTENANCE TREATMENT WITH LITHIUM

Tests that are commonly employed in the follow-up evaluation include periodic thyroid function testing (e.g., TSH), BUN, serum creatinine, and periodic ECGs. In medically stable patients, such follow-up evaluations might be done every six to 12 months. When concerned about potential lithium-induced renal toxicity, 24-hour urine volume, creatinine clearance, and protein excretion can be obtained. If the physical examination of the thyroid is abnormal, or the history is suggestive of thyroid disease, a more extensive thyroid function test panel should be obtained (e.g., add T_3, T_4).

LITHIUM BLOOD LEVELS

The utility of monitoring serum lithium levels in patients with bipolar mood disorder is well established. For acute mania, Jefferson et al. (12) suggested therapeutic lithium levels from a lower range of 0.8 to 1.0 mEq/liter to an upper range of about 1.4 to 1.5 mEq/liter. Amdisen (13) described a "warning range" between 1.2 to 1.5 mEq/liter, in which the risk of developing lithium toxicity begins to rise rapidly. Toxic reactions to lithium have been most commonly seen when the serum lithium level exceeds 1.5 mEq/liter. However, lithium toxicity has been observed in patients whose serum lithium levels were below the 1.2 to 1.5 mEq/liter range (14); this can especially be the case in elderly or medically ill patients. The therapeutic and toxic ranges for lithium are very close and at times might even overlap. Severe lithium toxicity is usually seen when serum lithium levels approach or exceed 3 mEq/liter. Lithium levels at 4 mEq/liter or more are typically regarded as a medical emergency. In the context of severe lithium toxicity, medical consultation is advised (e.g., to assess need for dialysis).

Stable, steady-state serum lithium levels are achieved after five half-lives for the lithium preparation used, which in individuals without renal dysfunction is usually about five to eight days after starting lithium or five to eight days after a dosage change. Nevertheless, it is sometimes recommended that lithium levels be checked a couple of times a week during the beginning stage of lithium therapy to help guard against lithium toxicity in patients who might require only small amounts of lithium to achieve therapeutic levels. This might be the case especially with older patients. Also, blood levels should be drawn in any patient demonstrating signs of possible lithium toxicity.

The currently accepted time to draw a serum lithium level is 12 hours after the last lithium dose (13). Values obtained in this manner can be meaningfully compared with the serum levels most commonly reported in the literature (the 12-hour post-lithium dose standard having been accepted internationally). However, in the context of severe lithium toxicity, more frequent lithium evaluations (e.g., every three hours) are sometimes used to follow lithium excretion and determine the need for dialysis (15). Dialysis is typically used in lithium-toxic patients with serum lithium levels greater than 4.0 mEq/liter or those patients with lithium levels between 2 and 4 mEq/liter with evidence of slow lithium excretion and poor medical status (see ref. 15). Although hemodialysis is useful in the removal of lithium from the body, rebound peaks in serum lithium concentration can occur after a session of hemodialysis. Medical specialists (e.g., internist, nephrologist) should be consulted in the case of serious lithium toxicity.

After resolution of an acute manic episode, maintenance therapy is generally prescribed at a lower lithium level than that required for the treatment of acute mania. Levels around 0.6 to 0.9 mEq/liter have commonly been advocated (12), although effective remission of affective symptoms has been reported at lower levels. For instance, Jerram and McDonald (16) reported similar relapse rates in bipolar patients with serum lithium levels less than 0.5 mEq/liter and in patients with higher levels (e.g., greater than 0.7 mEq/liter). Hullin (17) reported increased rates of relapse when the lithium levels fell to less than 0.4 mEq/liter. Prien and Caffey (18) reported that lithium levels of 0.8 mEq/liter or greater best protected against illness relapse. For elderly patients, levels between 0.4 and 0.7 mEq/liter have been described as effective (19). Despite being kept on the same lithium dose, serum lithium levels can rise when the patient is in a transition from an acute manic phase to some resolution of the mania (i.e., patients might need to have their dose lowered to prevent toxicity).

How low the clinician can go with a serum lithium level in certain bipolar patients and still achieve effective prophylaxis is an area of current investigation. Interestingly, there has even been a case report of effective treatment of a bipolar patient who was maintained at plasma lithium levels as low as 0.13 mEq/liter (20).

During maintenance lithium therapy, lithium levels are typically drawn on a periodic basis (e.g., every one to three months, or more or less often as clinically indicated). More frequent monitoring is indicated for patients with unstable renal function, patients undergoing dose changes of lithium, and patients taking or changing doses of medications that alter the renal excretion of lithium (e.g., diuretics and certain nonsteroidal anti–inflammatory agents such as ibuprofen). Different brands of lithium might have differing bioavailabilities; hence determining a lithium level after switching between different lithium brands or preparations is wise. Lithium level determinations are also indicated for patients who appear lithium toxic or are changing dietary salt intake, and during pregnancy and after delivery. (Lithium is contraindicated in the first trimester of pregnancy because of its association with congenital heart disease.) In patients at a maintenance blood level of lithium (e.g., 0.5 to 1.0 mEq/liter) who are showing early signs of redeveloping mania, lithium can be increased to achieve acute therapeutic levels (e.g., 1.0 to 1.4 mEq/liter).

EXPERIMENTAL METHODS OF MONITORING LITHIUM TREATMENT

Other proposed methods for monitoring lithium therapy include measuring salivary lithium levels (21, 22) or RBC/plasma lithium ratios (20). Measuring salivary lithium levels would be less traumatic and more convenient for the patient (i.e., it obviates need for more frequent blood draws). To use salivary lithium levels, each patient needs to have a ratio of saliva to plasma lithium determined so that the individual salivary lithium levels will be meaningful (23). On another note, investigators have searched for biologic markers predictive of lithium response. Higher RBC/plasma lithium ratios have been associated with bipolar patients who respond well to lithium (24); however, results in this area have been inconsistent (25). The utility of salivary lithium levels and RBC/plasma lithium ratios is still under study. The potential clinical value of these methods as either alternatives or adjuncts to serum lithium level monitoring awaits further clarification.

■ ANTIPSYCHOTIC MEDICATIONS

No universally accepted protocols exist for the pretreatment or follow-up medical evaluation of the patient on antipsychotic medications. Pretreatment laboratory tests are typically ordered as clinically indicated and include consideration of the patient's past medical history, results of the physical examination, previous history of adverse drug reactions, and knowledge of the potential adverse effects of the different antipsychotics (e.g., agranulocytosis, liver toxicity, ECG abnormalities). Agranulocytosis is perhaps most problematic with the antipsychotic clozapine; hence the frequent (e.g., weekly) periodic complete blood count (CBC) recommended by the manufacturer. For clozapine, most of the cases of agranulocytosis have been in the first four months of treatment, although cases occurring at a later time have been reported. Liver toxicity was most common in the past with chlorpromazine, and ECG abnormalities have been perhaps most associated with the antipsychotic thioridazine. Malignant arrhythmias have been reported in patients taking thioridazine, and patients who seem most susceptible to these arrhythmias are patients with preexisting prolonged QT intervals or those who develop prolonged QT intervals during treatment. Schwartz and Wolf (2) reported that when the corrected QT interval (QTc) exceeds 0.440 seconds, the risk is greatest for sudden cardiac death due to ventricular tachycardia or ventricular fibrillation. Patients with a history of cardiac pathology or prolonged QT intervals might need an ECG both before and during administration of an antipsychotic. Beresford et al. (26), however, argued that it is difficult to predict which psychiatric patients on any psychotropic medications will develop widened QT intervals. They suggested that the clinician needs to evaluate each patient on a case-by-case basis. This also applies to patients on TCAs.

As with the antidepressants, in the absence of a history of cardiac pathology, the clinician might order an ECG in a man over age 30 or a woman over age 40 who is about to be started on an antipsychotic associated with potential cardiotoxicity (e.g., thioridazine). Additionally, liver function tests should be ordered in patients with a history of liver disease who are about to be started on these medications. Finally, antipsychotics can be epileptogenic (especially chlorpromazine and thioridazine); patients with a history of a seizure disorder might need EEG follow-up.

NEUROLEPTIC MALIGNANT SYNDROME

Neuroleptic malignant syndrome (NMS) is a potentially fatal adverse reaction that can be seen in as many as 1 to 2.4 percent of patients on antipsychotic medication. Although antipsychotics have been implicated as the psychotropic medication most commonly associated with NMS, cases of NMS or NMS-like conditions have been reported 1) in patients taking other medications, such as monoamine oxidase inhibitors (MAOIs); 2) in patients taking tricyclic antidepressants, reserpine, meperidine hydrochloride, or prochlorperazine in combination with MAOIs; and 3) in situations where dopamine agonists, such as levodopa or amantadine, are suddenly withdrawn. NMS is often thought of as presenting with a tetrad of major symptoms: 1) hyperpyrexia, 2) autonomic instability (e.g., with blood pressure and pulse changes), 3) severe extrapyramidal dysfunction (e.g., rigidity, posturing), and 4) mental status changes of a delirious nature. Laboratory abnormalities that have been reported in this condition include creatine phosphokinase (CPK) elevations (in about 40 to 50 percent of NMS patients), leukocytosis (with a shift to the left) in about 40 percent of cases, myoglobulinuria, and occasional elevations in liver function tests. These abnormal values typically revert to normal on resolution of the syndrome. Complications of NMS can include aspiration pneumonia, respiratory arrest, acute renal failure, and cardiovascular collapse. Harsh (27) reported a case of NMS with a peak CPK elevation of 189,000 IU/liter. This patient also developed myoglobinuric renal failure (presumably from the significant muscle rigidity and subsequent muscle breakdown).

ANTIPSYCHOTIC BLOOD LEVELS

A number of techniques are available for the measurement of antipsychotics in patients' blood. These methodologies include gas-liquid chromatography (GLC), high-pressure liquid chromatography (HPLC), gas chromatography–mass spectrometry (GC-MS), fluorimetry, radioimmunoassay (RIA), and the radioreceptor assay (RRA) (28). Some of these techniques are able to detect only the parent drug compound; some detect the parent drug and a few metabolites. Others (e.g., RRA) are able to measure the activity of the parent drug as well as active drug metabolites. Although a large literature exists about the blood level measurement of various antipsychotics and their metabolites, no consistent therapeutic levels or clear therapeutic windows for any of the antipsychotics have been established. Indeed, the antipsychotic blood levels reported in patients with persistent psychotic symptoms tend to be very similar to the levels seen in patients in full remission. Also, the correlations between the prescribed neuroleptic dose and subsequent blood levels are not always very strong. However, low antipsychotic blood levels do tend to help identify those patients who are most likely to relapse (e.g., secondary to noncompliance or rapid metabolism of the neuroleptic for one reason or another). Preliminary work by Shostak et al. (29) suggested that levels of reduced haloperidol (a haloperidol metabolite) might better predict clinical response than levels of the parent compound.

The utility of antipsychotic blood levels is an area under investigation. Possible current uses might include 1) assessment of patient compliance, 2) assessment of patients taking their medications but achieving only very low and potentially ineffective blood levels, and 3) assessment of certain antipsychotic and other drug interactions. For example, Arana et al. (30) reported that carbamazepine can decrease the blood levels of haloperidol (e.g., through inducing hepatic enzymes), which can be associated with clinical deterioration. Silver et al. (31) noted that in two patients taking thioridazine and propranolol, the addition of propranolol caused as much as a fivefold increase in plasma thioridazine levels, making these patients more susceptible to toxicity from thioridazine (e.g., arrhythmias, pigmentary retinopathy). A similar increase in chlorpromazine levels has been noted in patients treated with both chlorpromazine and propranolol.

■ MONOAMINE OXIDASE INHIBITORS

In the patient on monoamine oxidase inhibitors (MAOIs), the laboratory tests that need the most careful attention are the liver function tests because these medications (especially the nonhydrazine MAOIs phenelzine and isocarboxazid) have been associated with (potentially fatal) hepatotoxicity. Additionally, some studies have reported that maximal therapeutic benefits of MAOIs (largely phenelzine) are obtained when the blood platelet monoamine oxidase (MAO) inhibition approximates or is greater than 80 percent (32). Results for phenelzine have been extrapolated by clinicians to other MAOIs (e.g., tranylcypromine). Whether the 80 percent inhibition level also applies to tranylcypromine has not been clearly established. The clinical usefulness of measuring blood platelet MAO inhibition for patients taking MAOIs will require further study.

■ ANTICONVULSANTS

Certain anticonvulsant medications (e.g., carbamazepine, valproic acid, clonazepam) are being increasingly utilized in the management of certain psychiatric conditions (e.g., bipolar disorders). A full discussion on the use of anticonvulsants in psychiatric illness is beyond the scope of this book. Our focus will be on two anticonvulsants for which the use of the laboratory is important: carbamazepine and sodium valproate.

A specific laboratory evaluation strategy for the anticonvulsant clonazepam has not been advocated. Clonazepam is a high-potency benzodiazepine that is being more frequently used by psychiatrists. In general, pretreatment or follow-up laboratory testing for patients taking any benzodiazepine for psychiatric reasons is not routinely recommended. However, for benzodiazepines requiring hepatic metabolism (e.g., clonazepam, chlordiazepoxide), elevated liver function tests might suggest a decreased capacity to metabolize the medication and hence a greater propensity to adverse side effects (e.g., sedation, dizziness, ataxia). Benzodiazepines themselves can also reportedly cause elevations in serum liver enzymes. Qualitative and quantitative blood and urine tests for the benzodiazepines are available, although they have not been shown to directly correlate with therapeutic efficacy.

ANTICONVULSANT BLOOD LEVELS

Therapeutic blood levels for anticonvulsants used in the treatment of psychiatric disorders have not been established. At this time, it is not clear if the therapeutic serum levels described as effective in epilepsy are also therapeutic for the psychiatric disorders these medications are being used to treat. However, Emrich et al. (33) supported using the therapeutic blood levels for carbamazepine and valproic acid that have been established for seizure control when using these medications in the treatment of mood disorders. On the other hand, at least for carbamazepine, Post (34, 35) suggested that the clinical monitoring of blood levels is probably only of secondary importance and that the therapeutic carbamazepine levels established for seizure control are not always applicable in the treatment of affective symptoms. However, Post et al. (36) suggested that blood levels of the -10,11-epoxide metabolite of carbamazepine might be related to therapeutic efficacy; others have suggested that this metabolite can contribute to certain neurologic side effects. The possible roles played by valproic acid metabolites such as 2-en valproic acid or 4-en valproic acid in the control of certain psychiatric symptoms is unclear at this time. Research in these areas continues.

For the anticonvulsants, a wide range of plasma medication levels can be found in patients on the same dose. Therefore, monitoring serum carbamazepine and valproic acid levels, and perhaps clonazepam levels, is important to the psychiatrist for predicting possible toxicity from these drugs. Side effects are generally more prominent when blood levels approach or exceed the upper limits of the established therapeutic ranges for seizure control. Additionally, blood level monitoring for the anticonvulsants is important when the patient is concomitantly taking certain medications known to affect the anticonvulsant blood level. For instance, medications that have been noted to be inhibitors of carbamazepine metabolism include erythromycin (and related antibiotics), isoniazid, verapamil, diltiazem, propoxyphene, cimetidine, nicotinamide, viloxazine, and valproic acid. Concomitant use of carbamazepine with any of these medications can potentially increase blood carbamazepine to toxic levels. Conversely, carbamazepine has enzyme-inducing properties and can lower the blood levels of certain other medications. Arana et al. (30) reported cases where carbamazepine seemed to lower haloperidol blood levels, with subsequent clinical deterioration. Carbamazepine can also reduce the steady-state levels of such medications as warfarin, doxycycline, ethosuximide, valproic acid, and clonazepam. On a final note, carbamazepine has the capacity to decrease its own blood level because of the medication's autoinduction property. Hence, a patient started and kept on the same dose of carbamazepine over a period of a month will commonly have a lower serum carbamazepine level at the end of the month than at the beginning of treatment.

The biologically active anticonvulsant compound is generally the medication or active metabolite that remains unbound to blood binding proteins such as albumin. Serum anticonvulsant levels typically measure total (bound plus unbound) serum concentrations. Usually, a total concentration is in direct proportion to the free concentration and is therefore a reasonable estimate of pharmacologic response (37). However, alterations in protein available for protein-binding can affect the meaning of a total serum anticonvulsant level, especially for carbamazepine, valproic acid, and phenytoin (38). Theoretically, decreased albumin concentrations can result in increased unbound fractions of these anticonvulsants, leading to perhaps an increased chance of toxicity, especially if the blood levels are kept in the upper range of therapeutic (therapeutic concentrations having been established for total serum anticonvulsants). Most "free" concentration ranges for the control of seizures that have been proposed have not been fully studied. Hence, for patients being treated with these anticonvulsants, it might often be useful to obtain some measure of the blood protein status (e.g., serum albumin level), especially when the level is suspected of being low (e.g., as in the case of patients with alcoholism, anorexia, significant weight loss, or protein malnutrition). Note that protein binding is not only reduced by hypoalbuminemia, but also by such conditions that alter the affinity of albumin for the anticonvulsant (e.g., through albumin configuration changes that can be seen in renal failure) or by conditions in which the competition for protein-binding sites is increased (e.g., by bilirubin or certain other drugs).

GENERIC VERSUS BRANDED ANTICONVULSANTS

It has been noted that when switching from a branded to a generic anticonvulsant (or vice versa) serum blood levels can vary because of differing bioavailabilities of the two medication preparations. It is recommended that switches between the branded and generic anticonvulsants be accompanied by some monitoring of the anticonvulsant blood levels for the first month or so (39). Adjustments in the medication dosage might be necessary to maintain therapeutic or nontoxic blood levels.

PRETREATMENT AND FOLLOW-UP OF PATIENTS TREATED WITH CARBAMAZEPINE

Table 8-3 lists some of the major components of a carbamazepine laboratory evaluation. Because of the possibility of hematologic changes in patients on carbamazepine, periodic

TABLE 8-3. **Suggested Pretreatment Carbamazepine Laboratory Evaluation**

- Complete blood count
- Platelet count
- Reticulocyte count
- Liver function tests
- Serum electrolytes (especially serum sodium)
- Electrocardiogram
- Pregnancy test in potentially childbearing women

follow-up of hematologic function is felt to be necessary. Table 8-4 outlines the type and frequency of hematologic toxicity that has been seen with carbamazepine. Besides a hematologic evaluation, other pretreatment laboratory and diagnostic evaluations include liver function tests, ECG, electrolytes, and a pregnancy test (when indicated). Baseline liver function tests prior to and sometime after carbamazepine is started should be obtained because of the risk of hepatotoxicity. The clinician should note that rare cases of fatal hepatic necrosis have been reported in patients taking carbamazepine (35); however, the incidence appears to be rare. Patients with abnormal liver function tests should have their liver function tests carefully monitored while on carbamazepine. Patients with a prior history of liver dysfunction might be more vulnerable to carbamazepine-induced hepatotoxicity.

An ECG is also usually obtained both before and during treatment because of the possibility of ECG changes similar to those seen with TCAs and phenothiazines (i.e., delayed cardiac conduction with QRS and QT prolongation). Patients with QTc intervals exceeding 0.440 seconds either before or during treatment are perhaps at increased risk of malignant cardiac arrhyth-

TABLE 8-4. **Hematologic Toxicity Associated with Carbamazepine**

Aplastic anemia:
  Prevalence: approximately 1/20,000 to 1/50,000
  Incidence: 0.5/100,000/year

Leukopenia (neutropenia):
  Prevalence
    Transient: 10 percent (range 2 to 60 percent)
    Persistent: 2 percent (range 0 to 8 percent)
  Average change: 0 to 1,000 per mm^3

Thrombocytopenia:
  Prevalence: 2 percent
  Average change: 0 to 20,000 per mm^3

Anemia:
  Prevalence: < 5 percent (range 0 to 10 percent)
  Average change: 0 to 0.5 g hemoglobin/dl

Note. From Hart RG, Easton JD: Carbamazepine and hematological monitoring. Ann Neurol 1982; 11:309–312. With permission.

mias (2). Additionally, as with the TCAs or phenothiazines, carbamazepine should be used cautiously in any patient with heart block. (Remember that carbamazepine is structurally similar to the TCAs and phenothiazines.) Cases of heart block associated with carbamazepine have been reported. Medications that interfere with the metabolism of carbamazepine (e.g., erythromycin) can increase carbamazepine blood levels into a range where cardiac toxicity becomes manifest.

Furthermore, serum electrolytes, especially serum sodium, should be evaluated periodically, especially if hyponatremia is suspected (e.g., in a patient with polydipsia or confusion). A few anecdotal reports of carbamazepine-associated hyponatremia and water intoxication have appeared in the literature. Some mild decreases in serum sodium, however, are not uncommon in patients on carbamazepine, and these small drops in the serum sodium (still in a "normal" range) are usually not clinically problematic. Vieweg et al. (40) reported less hyponatremia in patients treated with a combination of carbamazepine and lithium. Finally, carbamazepine might be teratogenic; hence, a pregnancy test is indicated in potentially childbearing women so that a full risk-benefit assessment can be made before starting or continuing carbamazepine.

EEG

Most psychiatric investigators do not feel that a normal EEG is a contraindication for using anticonvulsants such as carbamazepine in patients who are being given the anticonvulsant for some psychiatric indication. However, some clinicians have suggested that they might be more likely to consider using carbamazepine in the context of a patient with a history of epilepsy or some definite paroxysmal EEG abnormality, or even some nonparoxysmal EEG aberrations. Additional study looking for possible EEG or computerized EEG markers predictive of anticonvulsant response in psychiatric disorders is needed.

CONTROVERSIES SURROUNDING HEMATOLOGIC EVALUATION FOR PATIENTS ON CARBAMAZEPINE

Perhaps one of the greatest inhibitions psychiatrists have had in using carbamazepine for psychiatric indications has been the fear of hematologic complications, specifically aplastic anemia. Post (35) described an estimated incidence of aplastic anemia of around one in 20,000 to one in 40,000 patients.

The *Physicians' Desk Reference* (PDR) (41) suggests weekly hematologic evaluation for the first three months of carbamazepine therapy, and monthly follow-up thereafter for the first two or three years. Many psychiatrists and neurologists, including Hart and Easton (42), feel that such a laboratory testing strategy for carbamazepine is excessive and unnecessarily expensive. The hematologic follow-up Hart and Easton recommend is outlined in Table 8-5. The hematologic evaluation for patients who develop leukopenia while on carbamazepine is listed in Table 8-6. Additionally, a stat hematologic evaluation is indicated in any patient on carbamazepine who develops signs or symptoms of bone marrow suppression (e.g., petechiae, pallor, undue weakness, fever, or infection). Also, platelet counts might need to be checked prior to surgical procedures.

Minor decreases in the WBC count are common in patients taking carbamazepine. Post (34) suggested slightly different guidelines for carbamazepine discontinuation than did Hart and Easton (42); these include a WBC count less than $3,000/mm^3$, erythrocyte count less than $4.0 \times 10^6/mm^3$, hemoglobin less than 11 mg/dl, platelets less than $100,000/mm^3$, reticulocyte count less than 0.3 percent, and serum iron greater than 150 mg/dl. Somewhat more conservative hematologic thresholds for stopping carbamazepine administration provided by the manufacturer can be found in the PDR (41). Interestingly, at the other end of the spectrum of vigilance for hematologic complications in

TABLE 8-5. **Suggested Hematologic Follow-up for Patients Treated with Carbamazepine**

---

1. Do complete blood count every two weeks for first two months.

2. Barring abnormalities, count then can be obtained quarterly.

3. Watch for petechiae, pallor, undue weakness, fever, or signs of infection. In the event that any of these (or other) signs or symptoms of potential bone marrow suppression become manifest, an immediate hematologic evaluation (i.e., complete blood count) is indicated.

Note. Adapted from Hart RG, Easton JD: Carbamazepine and hematological monitoring. Ann Neurol 1982; 11:309–312.

TABLE 8-6. **Suggested Hematologic Evaluation in Patients Who Develop Leukopenia While on Carbamazepine**

1. Discontinue carbamazepine in presence of infection or severe leukopenia (less than 3000 white blood cells/mm³ or less than 1,500 neutrophils/mm³).

Otherwise:

2. Monitor every two weeks, waiting until return to baseline; however, might want to decrease carbamazepine dose.

Note. Adapted from Hart RG, Easton JD: Carbamazepine and hematological monitoring. Ann Neurol 1982; 11:309–312.

patients taking carbamazepine, Post (35) reported that many neurologists in England do no hematologic monitoring at all.

■ SODIUM VALPROATE

The anticonvulsant sodium valproate is also being utilized in certain psychiatric disorders, such as recurrent major mood (e.g., bipolar) and schizoaffective disorders (43). As with carbamazepine, therapeutic blood levels for the management of epilepsy have been established for valproic acid, but it is not known if these levels are also optimal for the management of psychiatric illness. However, some preliminary therapeutic levels for patients taking valproate for psychiatric conditions have been proposed by McElroy et al. (43) and are between 50 and 120 mg/liter (which coincides with typical therapeutic levels for seizure control). Indeed, most studies investigating the use of valproic acid in psychiatric illness have attempted to keep the patient in the therapeutic ranges established for seizure control. Levels exceeding the upper therapeutic limit for seizure control (typically between 100 and 120 mg/liter) are associated with greater chances of adverse side effects.

Some serious problems that have been associated with valproate include hepatotoxicity (ranging from mild hepatic dysfunction to fatal hepatic necrosis), hematologic abnormalities (e.g., thrombocytopenia, bone marrow suppression, leukopenia, anemia), and acute hemorrhagic pancreatitis. Mild elevations of serum transaminase levels (e.g., serum glutamic-oxaloacetic transaminase [SGOT]) are not uncommon. Risk factors for fatal hepatic necrosis seem to include young age (i.e., less than two years of age) and the taking of multiple anticonvulsants. A conservative laboratory testing strategy for patients on sodium valproate is outlined in Table 8-7. Additionally, elevated blood ammonia levels have been reported in patients on valproate in the absence of abnormal liver function tests. Valproate has also been associated with altered thyroid function tests (the clinical significance of which is unknown). Furthermore, valproate is partially eliminated in the urine as a ketometabolite, which can lead to a false-positive urine ketone test. This anticonvulsant is potentially teratogenic; hence, a pregnancy test should be obtained when indicated.

McElroy et al. (43) suggested that the presence of "nonparoxysmal EEG abnormalities" (e.g., generalized or localized slowing) might predict a favorable response to valproate. One of their bipolar patients who responded well to sodium valproate had brief bursts of high voltage sharp and slow activity. However, some of their patients who responded best had unremarkable EEGs.

■ ELECTROCONVULSIVE THERAPY

Certain laboratory and other diagnostic tests are typically ordered before a patient begins electroconvulsive therapy (ECT)

TABLE 8-7. **Suggested Blood Tests for Patients Receiving Valproic Acid or Its Derivatives**

- Complete blood count [a]
- Liver enzymes, bilirubin [a]
- Total protein, serum albumin
- Prothrombin time, partial thromboplastin time, bleeding time
- Serum level determination of concomitant antiepileptic drugs
- Thyroid function tests (especially if there is a history of thyroid disorder)
- Pregnancy test in potentially childbearing women

[a] Every two weeks for the first three months, then monthly for three months, then quarterly.

TABLE 8-8. **Evaluation Before Electroconvulsive Therapy**

- Complete blood count
- Blood chemistry panel
- Chest X ray
- Spinal X ray (if indicated)
- Urinalysis
- Electrocardiogram
- Computed tomography if indicated (see Table 7-1)

(44). A common "pre-ECT" workup is outlined in Table 8-8. A computed tomography (CT) scan and/or EEG can also be ordered when there are indications based on the history or physical, neurologic, or mental status examinations (see Table 7-1). Spinal X rays as part of the pre-ECT workup are currently less important because there is a lower incidence of orthopedic complications during the modern administration of ECT (largely due to the use of the muscle relaxant succinylcholine prior to ECT). However, patients with a history or physical examination suggestive of spine pathology might get X rays of the spine to search for areas of spine instability vulnerable to fracture or dislocation in case the administered muscle relaxant becomes ineffective during the ECT procedure.

Routine pre-ECT screening for abnormal serum pseudocholinesterase activity is not necessary except perhaps in the patient with a history of prolonged succinylcholine-induced apnea or in the patient with a blood relative with such a history. Elevations of serum CPK can also be seen in patients receiving ECT; however, brain-type CPK elevations are not seen (45).

■ REFERENCES

1. Gelenberg A: Laboratory tests for patients taking psychotropic drugs. Massachusetts General Hospital Newsletter Biological Therapies in Psychiatry 1983; 6:5–7
2. Schwartz P, Wolf S: QT interval prolongation as prediction of sudden death in patients with myocardial infarction. Circulation 1978; 57:1074–1077
3. Flugelman MYH, Tal A, Pollack S, et al: Psychotropic drugs and

long QT syndromes: case reports. J Clin Psychiatry 1985; 46:290–291

4. Boehnert MT, Lovejoy FH: Value of the QRS duration versus the serum drug level in predicting seizures and ventricular arrhythmias after an acute overdose of tricyclic antidepressants. N Engl J Med 1985; 313:474–479

5. American Psychiatric Association Task Force on the Use of Laboratory Tests in Psychiatry: Tricyclic antidepressants—blood level measurements and clinical outcome: an APA Task Force report. Am J Psychiatry 1985; 142:155–162

6. Siris SG: Schizophrenic woman on neuroleptic medication suffers secondary depression. Hosp Community Psychiatry 1988; 39:24–27

7. Lydiard RB: Desipramine in agoraphobia with panic attacks: an open, fixed-dose study. J Clin Psychopharmacol 1987; 7:258–260

8. Maarbjerg K, Vestergaard P, Schou M: Changes in serum thyroxine (T_4) and serum thyroid stimulating hormone (TSH) during prolonged lithium treatment. Acta Psychiatr Scand 1987; 75:217–221

9. Goodnick P, Fieve R, Schlegel A: Clinical and chemical effects of lithium discontinuation. Am J Psychiatry 1987; 144:385

10. Kutcher S, Gow S: Free T_4 measurement is preferred to the T_4 test for thyroid treated patients. Can J Psychiatry 1987; 32:112–114

11. Brady H, Hogan J: Lithium and the heart: unanswered questions. Chest 1988; 93:166–169

12. Jefferson JW, Greist JH, Ackerman DC: Lithium Encyclopedia for Clinical Practice. Washington, DC, American Psychiatric Press, 1983

13. Amdisen A: Monitoring lithium dose levels: clinical aspects of serum lithium estimation, in Handbook of Lithium Therapy. Edited by Johnson FN. Lancaster, England, MTP Press, 1980

14. Reisberg B, Gershon S: Side effects associated with lithium therapy. Arch Gen Psychiatry 1979; 36:879–887

15. Thomsen K, Schou M: The treatment of lithium poisoning, in Lithium Research and Therapy. Edited by Johnson FN. New York, Academic Press, 1975

16. Jerram TC, McDonald R: Plasma lithium control with particular reference to minimum effective levels, in Lithium in Medical Practice. Edited by Johnson FN, Johnson S. Lancaster, England, MTP Press, 1978

17. Hullin RP: Minimum serum lithium levels for effective prophylaxis, in Handbook of Lithium Therapy. Edited by Johnson FN. Baltimore, University Park Press, 1980

18. Prien RF, Caffey EM: Relationship between dosage and response to lithium prophylaxis in recurrent depression. Am J Psychiatry 1976; 133:567–570

19. Foster JR, Rosenthal JS: Lithium treatment of the elderly, in Handbook of Lithium Therapy. Edited by Johnson FN. Lancaster, England, MTP Press, 1980

20. Yassa R, Nair V, Kraus DJ: A possible indication for red cell lithium determinations: case report. Can J Psychiatry 1984; 29:44–45

21. Jefferson JW, Griest JH, Ackerman MS, et al: Lithium Encyclopedia for Clinical Practice, 2nd ed. Washington, DC, American Psychiatric Press, 1987

22. Ravenscroff P, Vozeh S, Weinstein M, et al: Saliva lithium concentrations in the management of lithium therapy. Arch Gen Psychiatry 1978; 35:1123–1127

23. Sims A: Monitoring lithium dose levels: estimations of lithium in saliva, in Handbook of Lithium Therapy. Edited by Johnson FN. Lancaster, England, MTP Press, 1980

24. Flemenbaum A, Weddige R, Miller J: Lithium erythrocyte/plasma ratio as a predictor of response. Am J Psychiatry 1978; 135:336–338

25. Frazer A, Gottlieb J, Mendels J: Lithium ratio and clinical response in manic depressive illness. Lancet 1977; 1:41–42

26. Beresford TP, Wilson F, Hall RCW, et al: Q-T prolongation in psychiatric outpatients. Psychosomatics 1986; 27:497–500

27. Harsh HH: Neuroleptic malignant syndrome: physiological and laboratory findings in a series of nine cases. J Clin Psychiatry 1987; 48:328–333

28. Creese I, Synder SH: A simple and sensitive radioreceptor assay for antischizophrenic drugs in blood. Nature 1977; 270:180–182

29. Shostak M, Perel JM, Stiller RL, et al: Plasma haloperidol and clinical response: a role for reduced haloperidol in antipsychotic activity? J Clin Psychopharmacol 1987; 7:394–400

30. Arana GW, Goff DC, Friedman H, et al: Does carbamazepine-induced reduction of plasma haloperidol levels worsen psychotic symptoms? Am J Psychiatry 1986; 143:650–651

31. Silver JM, Yudofsky SL, Kogan M, et al: Elevations of thioridazine plasma levels by propranolol. Am J Psychiatry 1986; 143:1290–1292

32. Liebowitz MR, Quitkin FM, Stewart JW, et al: Phenelzine versus imipramine in atypical depression: a preliminary report. Arch Gen Psychiatry 1984; 41:669–677

33. Emrich HM, Stoll KD, Muller AA: Guidelines for the use of carbamazepine and of valproate in the prophylaxis of affective disorders, in Anticonvulsants in Affective Disorders. Edited by Emrich HM, Okuma T, Muller AA. Amsterdam, Excerpta Medica, 1984

34. Post RM: Clinical approaches on the treatment resistant manic and depressive patient, in Psychopharmacology in Practice: Clinical and Research Update 1984. Bethesda, MD, Foundation for Advanced Education in the Sciences, 1984

35. Post RM: Clinical perspectives on the use of carbamazepine in manic-depressive illness. Psychiatry Letter 1985; 3:1–8

36. Post RM, Uhde TW, Ballenger JC, et al: Carbamazepine and its -10,11-epoxide metabolite in plasma and CSF. Arch Gen Psychiatry 1983; 40:673–676

37. Fitzsimmons WE: The role of metabolites and protein binding in antiepileptic monitoring. Resident and Staff Physician 1987; 33:151–159

38. Levy RH, Schmidt D: Utility of free level monitoring of antiepileptic drugs. Epilepsia 1985; 26:199–204

39. Sachdeo RC, Belendiuk G: Generic versus branded carbamazepine. Lancet 1987; 1:1432

40. Vieweg V, Glick JL, Herring S, et al: Absence of carbamazepine-induced hyponatremia among patients also given lithium. Am J Psychiatry 1987; 144:943–947

41. Physicians' Desk Reference: Oradell NJ, Medical Economics Company, 1986

42. Hart RG, Easton JD: Carbamazepine and hematological monitoring. Ann Neurol 1982; 11:309–312

43. McElroy SL, Keck PE, Pope HG: Sodium valproate: its use in primary psychiatric disorders. J Clin Psychopharmacol 1987; 7:16–24

44. Sakauye KM: A model for administration of electroconvulsive therapy. Hosp Community Psychiatry 1986; 37:785–788

45. Taylor PJ, Von Witt RJ, Fry AH: Serum creatine phosphokinase activity in psychiatric patients receiving electroconvulsive therapy. J Clin Psychiatry 1981; 42:104–105

APPENDIX A: SENSITIVITY, SPECIFICITY, AND PREDICTIVE POWER

Three concepts useful for an improved understanding of the meaningfulness of laboratory findings are sensitivity, specificity, and predictive power. These three terms are often used to describe the clinical value and validity of diagnostic tests. Not all patients with a particular disease will manifest all the laboratory abnormalities commonly associated with the disorder, and not all patients with the abnormalities will have the disorder. Therefore, presence or absence of a laboratory abnormality is not always definitive proof that a certain disorder is or is not present; it typically just increases or decreases the *probability* that the disorder is or is not present (some tests more so than others). Sensitivity, specificity, and predictive power help us in evaluating the predictive ability of a positive or negative finding. These values can vary among different populations of patients (e.g., general population versus hospitalized patients).

■ SENSITIVITY

Sensitivity is defined as the percentage of positive test results in patients who actually have the disease. The term describes the probability of a test being appropriately positive in a patient who has the particular disease in question. Therefore, a test with perfect sensitivity will detect all patients who have the disease. The sensitivity value is determined from the results of tests done on subjects with the disease. However, the sensitivity values for a particular test that are obtained in different patient populations might vary if the criteria for the disease were different.

The formula used to calculate sensitivity is

$$\frac{\text{true positives}}{\text{true positives} + \text{false negatives}} \times 100$$

Note that the denominator contains all the patients with the disease.

For instance, the sensitivity of the dexamethasone suppression test (DST) in depression has been estimated to be about 45 percent (perhaps higher in psychotic affective disorder). In other words, only about 45 percent of patients with diagnosable depression reportedly have a positive DST result (i.e., DST nonsuppression).

■ SPECIFICITY

Specificity is defined as the percentage of negative results among individuals who do not have the disease for which they are being tested. The term expresses the probability that someone who does not have the disease in question will have an appropriately negative test. Hence, a test with perfect specificity will be negative in all persons who do not have the disease (no false positives). Values for specificity are determined in populations of subjects free of the disease. Specificity values can vary between different populations. Specificity values might be high in a carefully screened disease-free control population, but lower when patients with conditions perhaps related to the disease in question are included.

The formula used to calculate specificity is

$$\frac{\text{true negatives}}{\text{true negatives} + \text{false positives}} \times 100$$

Note that the denominator contains all those individuals who do not have the disease.

For instance, the specificity of the DST in healthy, nondepressed persons is estimated to be approximately 90 percent. However, the specificity falls to 80 percent when the DST is used in patients with other psychiatric disorders (i.e., besides major depression). In this latter case, the number of false positives seems to increase.

■ PREDICTIVE POWER

The predictive power of a test result is defined as the percentage of results, values, and findings that are truly accurate. It describes the probability that a patient with a positive test actually has the particular disease, and the probability that a patient with a negative result truly does not have the disorder. A test with perfect positive predictive power will be positive only in those individuals who have the disease. A formula for the positive predictive value is

$$\frac{\text{true positives}}{\text{true positives} + \text{false positives}} \times 100$$

A formula for negative predictive power would be

$$\frac{\text{true negatives}}{\text{true negatives} + \text{false negatives}} \times 100$$

The denominators in these equations are not either all patients with the disease or all patients without the disease, but the numbers of patients with or without "abnormalities." Therefore, a positive predictive value helps the clinician assess the probability of a patient with a positive finding ("abnormality") actually having the disease; a negative predictive value helps the clinician assess the probability of a patient with a negative finding (i.e., "normal" finding) not having the disease.

APPENDIX B: SELECTED LABORATORY AND DIAGNOSTIC WORKUPS

What follows are lists of some commonly utilized laboratory and diagnostic tests for certain selected psychiatric conditions. Consensus about the tests included in these lists will vary. Other tests not included on these lists should be ordered as appropriate because different specific clinical situations will demand varying strategies. The clinician's choice of laboratory and other diagnostic tests should be individualized based on the patient's history and physical and mental status examinations.

■ ALCOHOL ABUSE AND DEPENDENCE

- Complete blood count (check the mean corpuscular volume and red cell distribution width)
- Serum electrolytes, glucose, blood urea nitrogen, creatinine
- Liver enzymes
  gamma-Glutamyl transaminase (GGT) (high sensitivity for recent alcohol abuse in a high-risk population)
  Aspartate aminotransferase (AST), also known as serum glutamic-oxaloacetic transaminase (SGOT)
  Alanine aminotransferase (ALT), also known as serum glutamic-pyruvic transaminase (SGPT)
  Alkaline phosphatase
- Total protein
- Serum albumin
- Prothrombin time
- Serum calcium and magnesium
- Serum uric acid
- Urine toxicology for other drugs of abuse
- Blood alcohol level
- Screening test for syphilis (Venereal Disease Research Laboratories [VDRL] or rapid plasma reagin [RPR])
- Electrocardiogram
- Chest X ray
- Urinalysis

- Stool for occult blood
- Plasma ammonia in patient with suspected hepatic encephalopathy
- Skull X ray and/or computed tomography scan in patient with previously unevaluated head trauma

■ ANOREXIA NERVOSA

Hsu (1) described a routine test battery that consists of

- Complete blood count
- Sedimentation rate; typically low in anorexia (1), can be useful in differential diagnosis. (However, because the sedimentation rate can be low in patients with infectious, inflammatory, or malignant disease, the use of the sedimentation rate here is controversial.)
- Liver function tests
- Tine test
- Chest X ray
- Electrocardiogram

Other commonly ordered tests (routine for some clinicians and supplemental for others) include

- Blood chemistry profile, including electrolytes and blood glucose (It would probably be wise to order this routinely, however, because electrolyte abnormalities can be a cause of death in anorexia nervosa.)
- Urinalysis
- Plasma cortisol levels
- Renal function tests (blood urea nitrogen, serum creatinine)
- Thyroid function tests
- Pituitary hormone levels
- Electroencephalogram
- Skull X ray (e.g., to rule out brain tumors, especially pituitary tumors). (Weinberger [2] recommended computed tomography.)
- Stool and urine tests for suspected laxative abuse (if available)

Additionally, bone X rays revealing reduced bone densities (osteopenia) have been reported in patients with anorexia nervosa.

■ ATYPICAL PSYCHOSIS

- Complete blood count with differential
- Serum electrolytes
- Blood glucose
- Renal functions (blood urea nitrogen (BUN), creatinine)
- Hepatic functions
- Blood calcium and phosphate
- Thyroid function tests
- Serum cortisol
- Screening test for syphilis (VDRL or RPR)
- Human immunodeficiency virus serology in potentially high-risk patients
- Vitamin B_{12} and folate levels in serum
- Urinalysis
- Urine toxicology (e.g., illicit drugs, heavy metals, anabolic steroids). Careful history to explore potential recreational, occupational, or residential drug/toxin exposure is important.
- Urine for uroporphyrins and porphobilinogen
- Chest X ray
- Electrocardiogram
- Sleep deprivation electroencephalogram (nasopharyngeal leads might be helpful)
- Computed tomography and/or magnetic resonance imaging scan

■ BULIMIA

- Complete blood count
- Serum electrolytes, glucose, blood urea nitrogen, creatinine
- Serum calcium, phosphate
- Serum amylase
- Electrocardiogram
- Urinalysis

- Urine toxicology screen for drugs of abuse (especially cocaine)
- Stool and urine tests for laxative abuse (if available)

■ DEMENTIA

LABORATORY AND DIAGNOSTIC TEST BATTERY FOR PATIENTS WITH NEW ONSET OF DEMENTIA (3; also see Table B-1)

- Complete blood count
- Electrolyte panel
- Screening metabolic panel (including liver function tests, BUN, serum creatinine)
- Thyroid function tests
- Vitamin B_{12} and folate levels in serum
- Screening test for syphilis (VDRL or RPR)
- Urinalysis

TABLE B-1. **Supplemental Studies as Recommended by the National Institutes of Health Consensus Conference on the Differential Diagnosis of Dementing Diseases**

Test	Indication
Computed tomography (without contrast)	History suggestive of central nervous system mass lesion Focal neurologic signs Dementia of brief duration
Electroencephalogram	Altered consciousness (e.g., delirium)
Magnetic resonance imaging	Can clarify ambiguous computed tomography findings
Lumbar puncture	Clinical findings suggest infection (e.g., meningitis) or vasculitis
Carotid ultrasound	Of no value except sometimes in search for the cause of infarcts

Note. National Institutes of Health Consensus Development Panel: Differential diagnosis of dementing disease. National Institutes of Health Consensus Development Conference Statement 1987; 6:1–9

- Electrocardiogram
- Chest X ray
- Serum electrophoresis included by some clinicians

■ **GENERAL PSYCHIATRIC PATIENT ADMISSION BATTERY (SELECTIVE) (4)**

- Complete blood count
- Serum thyroxine (T_4)
- Serum calcium
- Aspartate aminotransferase (AST), also known as serum glutamic-oxaloacetic transaminase (SGOT)
- Alkaline phosphatase
- Syphilis serology (VDRL or RPR)
- Urinalysis

Of course, other laboratory and diagnostic tests (e.g., serum electrolytes, urine toxicology screen, electrocardiogram) should be ordered as appropriate. Some clinicians advocate a more extensive admission battery (e.g., a full chemistry battery, including electrolytes, glucose, blood urea nitrogen, creatinine, serum proteins, calcium, phosphorus, liver enzymes, and a battery of thyroid function tests (5).

■ **NEUROLEPTIC MALIGNANT SYNDROME**

- Complete blood count
- Serum electrolytes, glucose, blood urea nitrogen, creatinine
- Creatine phosphokinase
- Urinalysis
- Urine myoglobulin
- Lumbar puncture if central nervous system infection suspected
- Workup (e.g., blood and urine cultures) for other causes of fever
- Electrocardiogram
- Chest X ray

■ REFERENCES

1. Hsu LKG: The treatment of anorexia nervosa. Am J Psychiatry 1986; 143:573–581
2. Weinberger DR: Brain disease and psychiatric illness: when should a psychiatrist order a CAT scan? Am J Psychiatry 1984; 141:1521–1527
3. National Institutes of Health Consensus Development Panel: Differential diagnosis of dementing disease. National Institutes of Health Consensus Development Conference Statement 1987; 6:1–9
4. Dolan JG, Mushlin AI: Routine laboratory testing for medical disorders in psychiatric inpatients. Arch Intern Med 1985; 145:2085–2088
5. Hoffman RS, Koran LM: Detecting physical illness in patients with mental disorders. Psychosomatics 1984; 25:654–660

APPENDIX C: LIST OF SELECTED ABBREVIATIONS

AACC	American Association for Clinical Chemistry
ACTH	adrenocorticotropic hormone
ADH	antidiuretic hormone
AEEGS	American Electroencephalographic Society
AEP	auditory evoked potential
AIDS	acquired immune deficiency syndrome
AIP	acute intermittent porphyria
ALA	δ-aminolevulinic acid
ALD	aldolase
ALT	alanine aminotransferase
ANA	antinuclear antibodies
Anti-HA	antibody to hepatitis A virus
APA	American Psychiatric Association
APTT	activated partial thromboplastin time
ARC	AIDS-related complex
AST	aspartate aminotransferase
AV	atrioventricular
BAL	blood alcohol level
BP	blood pressure
BSAEP	brain stem auditory evoked potential
BUN	blood urea nitrogen
$CaNa_2$ EDTA	calcium disodium edetate
CBC	complete blood count
CCA	chromated copper arsenate
CCK	cholecystokinin
CDC	Centers for Disease Control
CMV	cytomegalovirus
CNS	central nervous system
CNV	contingent negative variation
CO_2	carbon dioxide
CO_2T	total serum carbon dioxide
CPAP	continuous positive airway pressure
CPK	creatine phosphokinase
CRH	corticotropin-releasing hormone
CRP	C-reactive protein

CSF	cerebrospinal fluid
CSI	cortisol suppression index
CT	computed tomography
DCT	diurnal cortisol test
DDD-CT	double-dose delayed CT
DHEAS	dehydroepiandrosterone sulfate
DI	diabetes insipidus
DNA	deoxyribonucleic acid
DST	dexamethasone suppression test
EA	early antigen
EBNA	Epstein-Barr nuclear antigen
EBV	Epstein-Barr virus
ECG	electrocardiogram
ECT	electroconvulsive therapy
EEG	electroencephalogram
EIA	enzyme immunoassay
ELISA	enzyme-linked immunosorbent assay
EMG	electromyogram
EMIT	enzyme-multiplied immunoassay technique
ENG	electronystagmography
EOG	electro-oculogram
EP	evoked potential
ESR	erythrocyte sedimentation rate
FANA	fluorescent antinuclear antibodies
FBS	fasting blood sugar
FEP	free erythrocyte protoporphyrin
FSH	follicle-stimulating hormone
fT_3	free T_3
fT_4	free T_4
FTA-ABS	fluorescent treponemal antibody absorption
FTI	free thyroxine index, or FT_4 index
GC-MS	gas chromatography–mass spectrometry
GGT	gamma-glutamyl transaminase
GH	growth hormone
GLC	gas-liquid chromatography
GTT	glucose tolerance test
HAA	hepatitis Australia antigen
HAAg	hepatitis A viral antigen
Hb	hemoglobin
HBeAg	hepatitis Be antigen

HBsAg	hepatitis B surface antigen
HCG	human chorionic gonadotropin
Hct	hematocrit
5-HIAA	5-hydroxyindoleacetic acid
HIV	human immunodeficiency virus
HPLC	high-pressure liquid chromatography
HPT	hypothalamic-pituitary-thyroid
HT	Hashimoto's thyroiditis
HTLV-III	human T-cell lymphotropic virus-III
HVS	hyperventilation syndrome
IF	intrinsic factor
IFA	indirect fluorescent antibody
IM	infectious mononucleosis
IRMA	immunoradiometric assay
LA	lupus anticoagulant
LAV	lymphadenopathy-associated virus
LDH	lactate dehydrogenase
LDL	low-density lipoprotein
LH	luteinizing hormone
LSD	D-lysergic acid diethylamide
MAO	monoamine oxidase
MAOI	monoamine oxidase inhibitor
MCH	mean corpuscular hemoglobin
MCHC	mean corpuscular hemoglobin concentration
MCV	mean corpuscular volume
MDMA	3,4-methylene dimethoxy-methamine
MI	myocardial infarction
MID	multi-infarct dementia
MMT	mixed meal test
MRI	magnetic resonance imaging
MRP	movement-related potential
MSLT	multiple sleep latency test
MVP	mitral-valve prolapse
Nd	selective attention effect
NH_3	blood ammonia nitrogen
NMR	nuclear magnetic resonance
NMS	neuroleptic malignant syndrome
NP	nasopharyngeal
NPT	nocturnal penile tumescence
NREM	nonrapid eye movement

PA	pernicious anemia
PBA	protein-binding assay
PBG	porphobilinogen
PCP	phencyclidine
PDR	Physicians' Desk Reference
PEEG	pharmacoelectroencephalography
PINV	post-imperative negative variation
PMS	premenstrual syndrome
PSS	progressive systemic sclerosis
PT	prothrombin time
PTH	parathyroid hormone
PTT	partial thromboplastin time
RBC	red blood cell
RDW	red cell distribution width
REM	rapid eye movement
RF	rheumatoid factor
RIA	radioimmunoassay
RPR	rapid plasma reagin
RRA	radioreceptor assay
rT_3	reverse T_3
RU	resin uptake
SAT	symptomless autoimmune thyroiditis
SGOT	serum glutamic-oxaloacetic transaminase
SGPT	serum glutamic-pyruvic transaminase
SIADH	syndrome of inappropriate secretion of antidiuretic hormone
SLE	systemic lupus erythematosus
SSEP	somatosensory evoked potential
T_3	triiodothyronine
T_4	thyroxine
TBG	thyroxine-binding globulin
TCA	tricyclic antidepressant
THC	tetrahydrocannabinol
TIA	transient ischemic attack
TIBC	total iron-binding capacity
TLC	thin-layer chromatography
TRH	thyrotropin-releasing hormone
TRHST	thyrotropin-releasing hormone stimulation test
TSH	thyroid-stimulating hormone

UCP	urinary coproporphyrin
UFC	urinary free cortisol
VBR	ventricle-to-brain ratio
VCA	viral capsid antigen
VDRL	Venereal Disease Research Laboratories
VEP	visual evoked potential
VMA	vanillylmandelic acid
WBC	white blood cell

INDEX